Wakefield Press

ENDO DAYS

Comedian, journalist, teacher, radio presenter and cabaret per-former Libby Trainor Parker does a lot of things, but writing is her first love. She had her first piece published in the *Canberra Times* when she was eight years old (a clever little poem about being addicted to telly), which could very well have been her peak. Libby has had her work published across a number of magazines and online news outlets, such as the *Advertiser, The Barker Mag, Rip It Up*, and *On the Record*.

ENDO DAYS

Libby Trainor Parker

Wakefield
Press

Wakefield Press
16 Rose Street
Mile End
South Australia 5031
www.wakefieldpress.com.au

First published 2023
Reprinted 2025

Edited by Jo Case
Text designed and typeset by Jesse Pollard, Wakefield Press

ISBN 978 1 74305 777 3

NATIONAL
LIBRARY
OF AUSTRALIA
A catalogue record for this
book is available from the
National Library of Australia

CORIOLE
McLAREN VALE
Wakefield Press thanks
Coriole Vineyards for
continued support

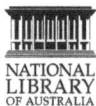

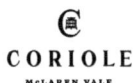

This book was written on the unceded lands of the Kaurna, Peramangk, Ngadjuri and Brayakaulung people. I pay my respects to Elders past, present and emerging. I acknowledge and pay respect to Traditional Owners of Country throughout Australia and recognise the continuing connection to lands, waters and communities. Always was, always will be
Aboriginal land.

Contents

Prologue ix

1 Knickers in a Twist 1

2 Endo 24

3 Ms Diagnosed 31

4 Managing your Endo 39

5 Endo and Mental Health 62

6 Coping with Endo 86

7 Endo Friendos, Support Groups
and Community 96

8 Chucking Sickies 118

9 Partners in Pain 146

10 Single with Endo 160

11 Parenting and Family Relationships
with Endo 167

12 Loss and Debacle 181

13 Endo Education 200

14 Remotely Helpful 210

15 Endo The Book 220

Endnotes 235

Acknowledgements 236

Prologue

Welcome to the Endo Days of your life!

One in nine people in Australia who menstruate have endometriosis, which is a progressive, chronic condition where cells similar to the lining of the uterus grow elsewhere in the body. These cells can grow on our organs, sticking them together, causing symptoms like – but not limited to – inflammation, chronic pain, fatigue, low mood, painful periods, painful sex, painful bowel and bladder movements, and fertility issues.

It's estimated that around 176 million people who menstruate worldwide are living with endometriosis, which means there are countless other people affected by the illness: patients have parents, partners, friends, colleagues, teachers, children, enemies, Uber drivers, baristas and . . . you get the picture. Hopefully, regardless of whether you are the protagonist or the co-star in the Endo Show, inside these pages you'll find something you can relate to, laugh at or reconcile with.

This book has been both a treasure and a trauma to write. When I was first approached with the idea of writing a long-form piece about my journey with a chronic health condition, I thought, *Sure! How hard could it be?*

I now have the answer to that. It's hard. And not just because my husband and I fostered a toddler at the same time as I was writing, so time and energy became very rare and extremely precious. But also, putting one's own stories out there feels like standing naked in a busy shopping mall, frantically waving your arms around while everyone else is gathered in front of you calmly sipping tea and wearing their Sunday Best.

But if there's one thing I know about chronic illness, it's that it can feel incredibly lonely. It can feel like everyone else in the whole world is getting on swimmingly with life and coping remarkably and you're the odd one out, because you're always two steps behind, running to catch up and feeling like no one will wait. It can feel like everyone around you is rolling their eyes at you, because 'it's always *something* with you, isn't it?' And it can be really tiring constantly explaining what's going on with your body and mind, especially if you aren't even sure yourself.

So, if you're reading this and you're living with a chronic illness or you're the supporter of someone living with a pain condition, know this: I see you. I hear you. You are not doing this alone. We're naked in the shopping mall together (okay, you don't have to be naked, but I just need some solidarity, you know?).

My stories are silly, sad, infuriating and sometimes inspiring. I'm not a doctor, so please see your qualified healthcare professional to discuss any of the strategies I mention in these pages. I'm writing this hoping that my tales will make you feel like we are all going through this together, whether you read them and shout, 'Yes! That's exactly like me!' or you think, *Ooh I'm so glad I don't have it like that.* We all want to feel better. Some of us don't even remember what it feels like to be well. And while there are plenty of great resources out there, there's always room for more, because the more we talk about endo and how we live our lives with it, the sooner the stigma will be lifted so we can be treated better, faster and with more dignity.

I have tried to use inclusive language where I can, but in some cases, like where I am quoting people verbatim, you will find some gendered language. Please forgive me for that. I have also included trigger warnings for content in some of the chapters, so skip past those if you need to keep yourself safe.

We all have an endo story to tell and mine isn't so different to others. I was diagnosed with endometriosis twenty-two years after first presenting with symptoms. The average diagnosis time these days is just under seven years. But if we talk more, tell our stories, support each other and stand up for ourselves, we can shorten that diagnosis time. Seven years is too long. We deserve to live well.

1

Knickers in a Twist

my endo story

Trigger warnings: *pregnancy loss, mental health*

As I emerged from my anaesthetic haze, two kind, concerned faces smiled down at twenty-one-year-old me. One face, which I discovered belonged to my surgeon, bore an uncanny resemblance to Ned Kelly, with wispy, waist-length hair and a full, bushy beard. The other face belonged to my father, who is far less bushranger-like.

'Do you want the good news or the good news?' Dr Ned asked in a gravelly (but friendly) voice. Without waiting for an answer, he continued excitedly, 'Your appendix is fine. Nothing wrong with it. It's a lovely, pink, squishy appendix.'

'What's the other good news?' Dad quizzed Dr Ned, who was looking mighty pleased with himself.

'I skilfully avoided cutting through that gorgeous tattoo.'

'Uh, tattoo?' Dad looked faint. My father, Phillip, is a kind and funny man with gentle eyes and a mischievous spirit. He's a drummer and an accountant, and I've always been really proud of him. He gave up playing drums when I was a toddler and then took it back up in his fifties. He now gigs around Sydney (Gadigal Land) like the total rockstar that he is. In fact, we've even played in bands together, which is one of the highlights of my life. Anyway, back to the whole Dad-discovering-I-had-a-tattoo thing.

An awkward silence followed as my father digested the information about my body art, which in 1999 was considered pretty risqué for ladies. I had it done out of pure early-twenties rebellion – but it's an adorable tiger cub lying on a purple orchid, so it doesn't exactly stick it to the man.

'So what's wrong with me?' I broke the silence. I was working at a ski lodge during the snow season and I had woken up with the worst pain I had ever felt. I walked, or rather, staggered to the local GP clinic and promptly collapsed on the waiting-room floor. I don't remember much about the ambulance ride to the nearest regional centre, just that all the nurses buzzing around me were pretty sure my appendix was inflamed and had to be removed immediately, lest it burst. I didn't even know what an appendix was. I've since learned it is a small, tube-shaped pouch attached to the large intestine and serves no real purpose.

'Yeah, probably a twisted bowel,' Ned growled in a sing-song way, which is quite a talent. 'Reckon you've got your knickers in a twist, mate.'

Dad snapped out of his post-tattoo-revelation shock to ask what our surgical bushranger meant by that. The answer has never left me.

'Oh, that's what it means when you're all upset about something: you've got your knickers in a twist. The saying comes from that feeling of lower abdomen pain because your bowel is twisted. That's what's wrong with you. You'll just need to find out what's got you in a tizzy and sort it out. Maybe quit your job.' And with a swish of his doctor coat, he bushranger-ed off to insult other patients.

Knickers? Tizzy? I thought. *Did I get taken in an ambulance all the way to another town for emergency surgery because I was all in a flap about something?* I was mortified. Was I certifiably insane?

I was born in Canberra (Ngunnawal country) and my family moved to Adelaide (traditional lands of the Kaurna people) when I was a teenager. I am still in Adelaide, where I live with my husband Matt, two stepdaughters, Niamh and Keeley, a little boy in our care, a very floppy cat called Hazel, a naughty cross-eyed kitten called Maui and a goldfish called Kylie Minnow.

At the 'appendix in a tizzy' stage of my life I'm discussing, though, I had run away to country New South Wales (traditional lands of the Ngarigo people) to work at a ski resort for the snow season, to get over a silly boy who absolutely did not deserve my heartbreak. Despite having no skills in skiing or snowboarding (nor body balance in general), the move was working wonders. I was having a great time, I'd pretty much forgotten about the silly boy and I was working hard and saving money with the intention of moving to Sydney (Gadigal land), where my dad lived, at the end of the season. I was meditating, reading lots of books, getting out to see stacks of live music, making questionable but fun romantic choices with tourists. Life was good. Why would my knickers have been in a twist?

Once I was discharged from hospital and started to make my way back to my snow digs, I had to decide whether to tell my housemates and workmates that there was actually nothing wrong with my appendix, that I'd had a significant surgery for no reason – and that I was actually, quite possibly, extremely unhinged, in the clinical sense. Dr Ned didn't perform keyhole surgery; he opened me right up. So, I still, to this day, have a very impressive scar next to my adorable, rebellious, tiger cub orchid.

My flatmates welcomed me back home, made me comfortable, propped me up with cushions and gave me cups of tea.

'Tell us all about it,' Suzie the ski instructor from Lake Tahoe urged, putting a rug over me.

'Oh it was awful,' I moaned. 'Damned appendix was ready to burst!' And then I unapologetically bathed in their sympathy for a while.

It wasn't the first time I was told the pain was in my head and it certainly wouldn't be the last.

Two years prior, at nineteen years old, I lived in Queensland (Yirrganydji territory) and worked in room service at a hotel casino. After dropping out of high school due to fatigue, low mood and zero motivation (I would later discover these were symptoms linked to my endometriosis and my recently diagnosed ADHD, which I am now medicated for and holy moly has it made a difference to my life!), I studied hospitality and worked in bars, clubs and hotels for years, before gaining adult entrance into university to study teaching.

I started teaching in 2006, and I completed a post graduate qualification in journalism in 2012. Teaching is fun, but very de-manding and physically taxing. After ten years of full-time teaching, I had to chuck it in because I simply wasn't well enough to do a good job anymore. I was letting my students down and they deserved better. I work for myself now, as a professional writer, and I take short-term teaching contracts when I am well enough and able to. Back when I was in hospitality, though, I travelled around a fair bit – trying to get that kink out of my twisted knickers, perhaps? At the time I ventured to Queensland (it was 1997, I reckon), I had been feeling flat, heavy, miserable and in pain on most days of the month, taking far too many days off work. I complained about it to a new pal at work one night.

'I think you have endometriosis,' she said. 'I was just diagnosed with it and all your symptoms sound exactly like mine.' Then she sashayed away (on rollerskates) to the high-rollers room in her Marilyn Monroe costume. (Her job was far more interesting than mine.)

'Endo-what-now?' But she'd already rolled to the rollers. I was left trying to remember what she'd said.

These days I know endometriosis is a condition where lining that is similar to the lining of the uterus grows in places it shouldn't, causing symptoms like pain, inflammation, fatigue, low mood and much more. The reason they say it's lining *like* that of the uterus is because it looks similar under a microscope, but isn't exactly the same. These words are all completely familiar now. But back then,

I couldn't even pronounce endometriosis, let alone describe my symptoms to the GP I took this information to.

'I have Endimeningitis,' I attempted, as a young-ish, handsome but stony-faced doctor stared back at me. 'Endo-elephantitis? Endomeningococcal??'

'You mean endometriosis,' he snarled. 'And you don't have it. You're just homesick. Endometriosis is a menstrual disease and you told me your periods aren't regular, so it can't be that. You need to stop partying, eat better and drink more water.'

'But I have all the same symptoms as my friend?'

'And where did you both get your medical degrees from?' he shot back at me. 'Don't come in here and diagnose yourself. You're fine. You're homesick and you need to ease off the nightclubs. Maybe get a new job.'

Look, he wasn't completely wrong. I had been working my way through every cocktail and bar snacks menu in Far North Queensland. But he didn't need to be so short with me. He didn't examine me, or ask about my pain. He didn't even touch me, nor refer me to a gynaecologist. He didn't prescribe anything to help (except sobriety); but on the upside, he was a firm contender for the National Eye-Rolling Championships, if that ever becomes a thing.

After several more visits to doctors over the years with complaints of back pain, abdominal pain, wild hormones, fainting, nausea, low mood and low immunity (and not a single referral to a gynaecologist), I am the proud owner of a list of diagnoses (and potential diagnoses) of many things that aren't endometriosis.

Highlights include: IBS (irritable bowel syndrome), bipolar, general anxiety disorder, viral meningitis, chronic fatigue syndrome, manic depression, Crohn's disease, polycystic ovarian syndrome, possible bowel cancer, appendicitis, stress, unexplained virus that just needs bed rest.

Here's a comprehensive list of things I *don't* have: bipolar, chronic fatigue syndrome, manic depression, Crohn's, appendicitis, polycystic ovarian syndrome, bowel cancer, unexplained virus that just needs bed rest.

Things I *do* have: endometriosis, adenomyosis,[1] premenstrual dysphoric disorder (PMDD),[2] fibromyalgia,[3] arthritis, stress (when I take on too much, which is often). I also did have viral meningitis for a spell in 2007.

Things I wish I'd had back in the mid to late 90s through to my diagnosis in the mid 2010s: knowledge about my body, awareness of (female) biology, education and empowerment. Also, doctors who didn't just see me as an over-dramatic, hysterical little girl who just needed to calm down, have two paracetamol, a glass of water and a good lie-down.

At the time of writing, diagnosis of endometriosis takes just under seven years (6.8 to be precise). And when I asked the Australian online endo community, they gave me this extensive list of ailments they were told they had or might have had before their eventual endo diagnosis (some of these people were teenagers at the time and many were regularly presenting to the emergency department when they received these diagnoses):

Pelvic infection, reflux, fibromyalgia, chronic pelvic inflammatory disease, depression, constipation, oversexed/sexually

---

1   Adenomyosis is a gynaecological condition where the lining of the uterus (endometrium) invades into the muscle of the uterus (myometrium). There are two types: it is called an 'adenomyoma' if only a section of the muscle is involved, and 'diffuse adenomyosis' when all the uterine muscle is involved. https://embracefertility.org/what-the-ouch-is-adenomyosis/
2   Premenstrual dysphoric disorder (PMDD) is a severe form of PMS that causes psychological distress and socioeconomic dysfunction. PMDD affects about 3-8% of women with PMS. https://www.jeanhailes.org.au/health-a-z/periods/premenstrual-syndrome-pms
3   Fibromyalgia is a common condition in which people experience symptoms that include widespread pain and tenderness in the body, often accompanied by fatigue and problems with memory and concentration.Fibromyalgia affects two to five per cent of the population, mainly women, although men and adolescents can also develop the condition. It tends to develop during middle adulthood. https://www.betterhealth.vic.gov.au/health/conditionsandtreatments/fibromyalgia

transmitted infection ('you've contracted an STI like gonorrhoea or chlamydia, probably from your boyfriend – is he cheating perhaps?'), pregnant, exaggeration ('it's just a bad period, take some Panadol and relax'), drug hunting/junkie, shingles, paranoia and anxiety ('there's nothing wrong with you, it's all in your head and you need a psychologist'), Crohn's, UTI (urinary tract infection), eating disorder, just feeling a bit crap ('hmmm sounds like a virus – go home and get some rest'), blood-clotting disorder, IBS ('it's a food intolerance of some sort. Start eliminating things from your diet today'), suspected bowel cancer, gallbladder issues, appendicitis, diverticulitis, womanhood ('it's just your body getting ready to have a baby, sweetheart'), Coeliac disease, lazy and unmotivated ('it's very clear to me and your parents you are faking being unwell to get out of school'), mood disorder, bipolar, stress, unfit, puberty, OCD, health anxiety, kidney stones, pancreas failure, heavy drinking ('sounds to me like a hangover – best have a Berocca and sleep it off'), stomach ulcer ('sounds like abnormally large veins pumping blood to the uterus, which is nothing to worry about'), gastroenteritis, RSI (repetitive strain injury), low pain tolerance, epilepsy. And my personal favourite: 'fat and constipated'.

Phew! What a list!

A special mention must go to the woman whose doctor told her to 'have an affair, because that would spice up your life and make you want to look after yourself better, which would make you lose weight and cure your pain'. Spoiler: it doesn't work like that. Exercise and a balanced diet can certainly have an impact, but the fat-shaming and dismissing of chronic pain patients with 'just dump the chub and you'll be right as rain' is not constructive. Fit people have endo pain, as do thin, curvy, overweight, underweight, and average-sized people.

It needs to be said that having an endo diagnosis doesn't mean you can't have any or all of the other things. In fact, endometriosis patients are known to have co-morbidities such as irritable bowel syndrome and overactive bladder syndrome; and anxiety and depression are common in people living with chronic pain and illness, so a mental health diagnosis isn't that unusual, nor is it completely unhelpful. Any time and energy you can put into improving your mental health is a win.

Chronic pain is pain that occurs long past the time it should take for healing from surgery, trauma or illness. It has been shown that rates of depression and psychological distress are higher among people with chronic pain than people without pain. According to Pain Australia, 'almost a third of Australian adults with severe or very severe pain experience high levels of psychological distress; around three times the rate of those with mild pain and six times the rate of those with no pain . . . suicidal behaviour is two to three times higher in people with chronic pain than the general population.'[4]

Finding a pain psychologist to join your endo cheer squad (your team of health professionals and supporters) is a fabulous idea and one I highly recommend. Pain can be traumatic, so try to look after yourself and keep yourself safe.

It also needs to be said that I certainly don't know everything and I am well aware that doctors can't know everything either. GPs have a tough job. They have to deal with everything from warts to whooping cough, colds to cancer. It's definitely not easy for them. That's why it is so important for us to arm ourselves with information that makes us able to look a doctor in the eye and say, 'I need your help and these are my symptoms'. And we need to couple that with zero tolerance for dismissive, belittling behaviour from doctors who should be helping us, not rolling their eyes.

I wish I had been more empowered and understood my body a

---

4   https://www.painaustralia.org.au/media-document/blog-1/blog-2020/blog-2019/
what-you-need-to-know-about-pain-and-mental-health-in-australia

little better when I was younger, and I wish I hadn't felt so alone. With all my diagnoses of mental illness, partying too hard and being told that if I quit my jobs I'd be happier and my pain would disappear, I poured all my energies into fixing a head that wasn't sick – which made my head a bit sick.

I felt isolated and stranded. I felt helpless, often. My body hurt so much and I was so tired, but there was no reason for it. My family thought I was just perpetually unreliable and over-dramatic, rather than chronically ill and struggling to stay afloat. I often felt like I was trying to breathe underwater. I became overtly extroverted in public as a mask and withdrawn and angry in private. I locked my emotions down and stopped trusting people because I didn't think I could trust myself. If I was so unstable that my brain was inventing all these physical issues, then I must be a danger to myself and those around me. I was not a good friend to others, nor myself.

When I look back at all the times I berated myself for being un-well, I feel frustrated and sad. What a waste. I could have been doing so many wonderful things and I could have been far more kind to myself for two decades. My relationships would have been better: I might not have chosen destructive and abusive partners, thinking that was all I deserved because I was a fuck-up. I might have even finished high school. Who knows? I am often angry when I think about it, because it could have been solved with kindness when I first asked about 'endimeningitis'. My doctor could have laughed at my mispronunciation (I wouldn't have minded!) and then said, 'Let's get you off to a gynaecologist to see what's going on there'. Imagine that.

There's a dark hangover from these experiences of mine, because I still doubt myself when I am ill. I am hesitant to seek medical assistance when I really need it, because I am so used to being turned away by doctors citing stress, anxiety and lack of job satisfaction.

Even during the Covid-19 pandemic, I was hesitant to go and get a PCR swab. I am so used to being eye-rolled and dismissed that I felt sure I'd be wasting everyone's time. Of course, I put that aside to do my civic duty. But the constant fear of being turned away and treated like I am a hypochondriac who is a burden rendered me disillusioned, frustrated and lacking in the confidence to speak up about my body. (The rejection sensitive dysphoria[5] or RSD I have – which is what it sounds like, an intense sensitivity to rejection, whether perceived or real – doesn't help.)

These days, I can pronounce 'endometriosis' and I am working on my trust issues. I am still happily extroverted, and now it's on purpose. But my lack of knowledge in my youth meant it took until I was thirty-six years old for a proper diagnosis. And by then, the damage to my body was significant.

We're all in this together: even the experts are learning as they go

My friend and colleague, Adelaide gynaecologist and endometriosis and fertility expert Professor Louise Hull, knows her stuff when it comes to endo. A smart, warm woman with a gentle New Zealand accent, Louise works hard for the endo community by keeping abreast of all the latest technology, treatment and innovation. If there's a conference, she's there. If there's news, she's all over it. If there's a new method for helping people with endo, she'll try it.

Like me, though, she often reflects on what could have been when she was younger and how things could have been better. She says it wasn't just patients who had a lack of knowledge. As a beginning gynaecologist, she and her peers didn't have the information they do now – but with new research and knowledge, she now sees things from different perspectives.

'If I could do anything differently to when I was a young gynae, I would ask much more careful questions about different symptoms,

---

5   Rejection sensitive dysphoria (RSD) is an emotional dysregulation that produces an extreme response to an actual or perceived rejection. It is often, but not always, connected to ADHD.

and I would do it in the context, not of trying to rush to a diagnosis of endo, but to think about whether it might be endo and if surgery might need be involved.'

Surgery isn't a cure for endometriosis. It's only one part of a treatment plan, which might consist of pain management, medication, pelvic physio, psychology and nutrition. Louise says she wishes she'd spent more time helping her patients through the brain's involvement with pain, like central sensitisation.

Central sensitisation is where the body is hypersensitive to things that aren't typically painful, but have become overactive due to high reactivity, which can prolong the pain. In short, your organs hurt and your nerves are over-reactive, so your brain tells everything to hurt. For an incredibly impressive and complex organ, the brain can also be a total jerk.

'We should have been asking more about pelvic sensitisation, somatic sensitisation – as in sensitisation of the muscles – and then central sensitisation, as well as bowel function, and be looking to treat in independent ways,' Louise admits. 'I would just be a lot more holistic about how to treat it. Not just thinking, *Well, I'll fix the endo by doing the surgery.* That's what we were certainly taught; that if there was endo there and you took it away, it was fixed. People really didn't understand the neural activation, but also the fact that your bowel could be affected, or your bladder, and that those symptoms needed treating by gynaecologists, not just, *Well, that's someone else's problem.*'

When she's talking about the pain and frustration endo patients lived with before doctors started taking a more holistic approach, Louise looks away and her eyes start to moisten. It's a hard conversation for both of us. But it's important for us to remember we're on the right track now and we're doing everything we can to improve life for people living with pain.

And these days, thankfully, more research is being focused on how stimulated nerve pathways in the colon, bladder and uterus can contribute to co-morbidity or make existing conditions worse through cross-organ sensitisation. With so many patients presenting with so many of the same symptoms and associated ailments, it has now become clearer that these things are often all part of the same condition. But that hasn't always been the understanding.

'I'm much more individualised with my treatment now,' she says. 'The central sensitisation, the fatigue and the headaches, also the mood and symptoms you get when you can't do stuff; they can actually give you three or four different diagnoses. But a lot of people don't even ask about those symptoms. Certainly, I didn't when I started, and I didn't recognise them as being part of the disease,' Louise says.

It was thirty years ago when Louise was just starting out, but she is now leading research teams that are working incredibly hard to make advances in endometriosis and uterus health in general.

'Back then, we didn't know very much about neural, we didn't know much about pain, and we couldn't measure nerves; we couldn't image brains. We didn't really understand the pain pathways,' she says.

So, what did that mean for those who were diagnosed or treated back then? People like me? Louise regrets that they might have been dismissed, or approached as though they had less resilience than others.

'I think they often weren't diagnosed, and there was an attitude of, *Everybody else has a period, but you can't take it, so therefore it must be a mental health thing.* I think, probably, as more female doctors came through, there was less of that, and it was better recognised that it wasn't quite right,' she says.

But it's not just doctors who give us the old, 'Toughen up, princess, it's just a period,' kind of mindset. Sometimes our mothers, grandmothers, sisters and aunties pass it down. Research shows endometriosis has a genetic disposition, which makes some people with a uterus more likely to get it than others. And because period health is a topic that has been taboo for a long time, misinformation can spread. In families like mine, it was thought that extreme pain, fainting, nausea and sick days were all part and parcel of being a person with a period.

The first time I got my period, at fourteen years old, I fainted and hit my head on the bathroom vanity on the way down. My mum and sister knew straight away it must be period pain, because they suffered the same. As I lay there on the cold tiles (which are amazing when you are feeling rotten, even in icy Canberra where I grew up), the women in my family shared their tales of woe about their cycles: the pain and the horror and the fainting and the nausea. I was mortified.

I counted the months until menopause (approximately 492, for the record) and it all seemed pretty bleak. I wondered how women had survived throughout the centuries and why they weren't permanently wearing helmets or protective gear to guard their heads from all the fainting. If this happened to all of us, how did the human race even exist? How did anyone get anything done?

I didn't have a very regular cycle in the beginning, but it was painful. My mum and sister were the same. My mum's mum the same as well. Mum told me my grandmother was dependent on painkillers. She died far too early, from heart failure at age fifty-two. I think I can assume the women in my family had undiagnosed endometriosis. That's why my mum told my sister and me that our pain was normal: because her mum had told her that, and probably Mum's mum's mum too.

My mother, Lorraine, is a clever, softly spoken woman who is one of the most tender and measured people I know. The polar opposite of me, she is shy, diplomatic and thinks before she speaks. (I'm not sure what happened to me.)

During my great menstrual revelations of 1992, Mum told me she missed at least two days of school every single month as a teenager. That's over 120 missed days of school. When she went to uni and then into work, she just learned to suck it up and breathe through the pain, like so many of us do. For some people who menstruate, pregnancy can stop the pain. So there are some medical professionals who will tell you that pregnancy stops endo and endo pain. After my mum had me, she said she didn't have the more significant symptoms anymore. So, I think we know what the cure for endometriosis is.

It's me. I'm the cure.

Kidding. There is no cure.

(Anecdotally, some people have fewer symptoms after pregnancy, but telling someone pregnancy will cure it is a big, steaming pile of horse shit.)

Despite plenty of evidence to the contrary and notwithstanding the knowledge that endo can cause fertility issues, the myth still seems to be floating around that people can be cured of endo if they fall pregnant. Regardless of their age, endo sufferers are being told to have kids even when they're not ready to, only to find that it does not, in fact, cure it at all.

And that myth is even worse for those of us who have had fertility struggles. If reading about pregnancy loss brings up difficult things for you, please consider skipping this next part to keep yourself safe.

Diagnosis is therapy: finally solving the pain puzzle

My first pregnancy loss was in 2013. It was heartbreaking – and it was actually how I received my diagnosis for endometriosis. Unfortunately for me, it was the first of eleven pregnancy losses, with no surviving pregnancies.

My first, much-wanted pregnancy was ectopic and grew on the outside of my uterus (a cornual ectopic) where it sat and rotted, causing significant decay of the corner my womb for about nine weeks. The pregnancy had been horrifically painful since I discovered I was expecting. But because I'd built a high tolerance for pain, I just breathed through it and endured. I just thought all pregnancies must be this painful. Again, I wondered how the human race continued to reproduce or get anything done, but I didn't want to bother anyone by going to the doctor, because I felt certain they would just eye-roll and send me on my way.

But one afternoon when I was sitting at my computer at work, clucky over my slightly swollen belly and ordering a baby bath and adorable onesies, I started to bleed. It was only the tiniest amount of blood, but it scared me. My colleagues told me I was fussing over nothing, that it would all be okay – but that I should get a scan to ease my mind. I went straight to the GP. When he touched my abdomen, I nearly jumped off the table. He gave me a look that told me I wasn't fussing over nothing and sent me straight to emergency, where they couldn't see a pregnancy in the uterus. The nurse asked me if I was even pregnant, which triggered that feeling that everything (even a pregnancy) was all in my head and I was wasting everyone's time. They did a pregnancy test and then let me know that, yes, I was definitely pregnant (what a relief?), but then a formal and extremely painful internal scan determined it was ectopic – but a rare kind of ectopic that made the hospital staff tilt their head at me in pity, and also want to have a good look because they'd never seen something like it before. I was very quickly scheduled for emergency caesarean surgery to remove my failed pregnancy, as well as the corner of my uterus.

After that surgery, and the long and heartbreaking recovery that followed, I was in excruciating pain most days of the month and my periods were longer and heavier than ever. I kept going back to my surgeon to ask if I was still decaying. Or was there an infection? Did he perhaps leave his scalpel in me? Could I be birthing an alien that implanted in me while I was under anaesthetic? Was I the antichrist and needing an exorcism, stat?

Each visit, I was sent away with Buscopan or Panadeine Forte and an explanation that I was 'just healing', 'maybe stressed?', 'probably grieving', and should 'maybe quit your job'. We had another contender for the National Eye Rolling Championships.

Then, finally, after twelve months of asking him to help me, my surgeon reluctantly agreed to do a laparoscopy, despite being 'absolutely sure there was definitely nothing wrong' with me. In fact, he was so convinced he wouldn't find anything wrong with me, when I walked into surgery, he was kicked back, relaxing on a chair with his feet up on the operating table (where I was about to lie), scrolling through his iPad and chuckling about . . . possibly cat videos? I dunno. He looked annoyed I was there. He looked annoyed *he* was there.

But after the surgery came the miracle: the reckoning. <Insert fanfare> *The Diagnosis*! Dr iPad came bounding into my hospital room with his treasured tablet. He was so excited. He said it was a hugely complex endometriosis case, especially the bits on my ureters spreading up to my kidneys. He enthusiastically flicked through all the photos of my messy insides on his iPad as he spoke like a giddy schoolboy about how amazing it was that the endo had snuck into so many nooks and crannies. It was equal parts gross and fascinating. But at least I finally knew what was wrong with me.

I wasn't making it up.

I wasn't a drama queen.

I didn't have to quit another job.

It wasn't a ploy for attention.

I was genuinely sick. And I had been right about my body for more than twenty years.

The relief of a diagnosis is monumental. It's as if a door, locked for so long, is finally opened, allowing you to walk through to the other side. There are challenges behind that door, but at least you can see them now and can learn how to manage them.

Now that I'm on the other side of the door, it's so important to me to open it for others. And despite my anecdotes and snarky sarcasm, I truly don't think doctors are to blame for every misdiagnosis. Like Louise says, the information and conversation just hasn't been available, or even acceptable. But as the good professor explains, there is now a greater community of specialists, GPs, patients, partners, and cheer squads, as well as a far better-educated generation of young people coming up. This gives us all so much hope.

'Young people now are more self-determined. When you give them control over their condition, diagnosis, and information, they do make good choices that are right for them,' Louise says. 'They're not scared of the topic of endo or knowing about their reproductive system. I think they're a lot more confident with those discussions. The more information we can give them, the earlier, the better.'

Once I had my diagnosis and spent some time grieving and aimlessly traversing the wild lands of Facebook groups and Doctor Google, trying to find what the hell I should do next, I'd quit my teaching job (the physical demands were no longer possible to withstand with the amount of chronic pain I was living with) and I started working in South Australia's state parliament for Greens member of the Legislative Council, Tammy Franks. She and I decided to move a motion asking for action on endometriosis in the form of an education program. I needed to do something so future generations wouldn't go through what I had and Tammy wanted to do something to help the countless people who had suffered with the illness without anyone to speak for them.

'Endometriosis was an issue that had been overlooked for far too long; unsurprisingly, because it was a women's health issue and most politicians have historically been men,' Tammy says. 'I was keen to help raise awareness and get real action because there are real people living with the condition, who are part of the statistics which are too often ignored. And the statistics are overwhelming. It was an honour to represent people with endo to start to make a positive change.'

So we wanted to do something. But I didn't know what. It just so happened at the time, there was movement at the station.

Where to from here: making lemonade from lemons

I'd heard of a group called Pelvic Pain Foundation of Australia (PPFA) who also wanted to educate young people about endo and period pain. As a teacher, I had connections in education and knowledge of how to put together learning resources. As a person working in parliament, I had access to people who could help us fund and advocate for a program, and, as an endo patient who waited a long time for a diagnosis, I could share what I wished I'd known twenty-two years earlier.

We were successful in securing support for the project, and chair of the PPFA board Associate Professor Susan Evans and I joined forces to create PPEP Talk® (Periods, Pain and Endometriosis Program) to roll out in South Australia and then across the country, as part of the National Action Plan for Endometriosis that Federal Health Minister Greg Hunt championed in 2017.

PPEP Talk® is a fun, fact-based program that empowers and educates secondary school students about period pain and endometriosis. I have since moved on from my involvement in the program and its organisation, but I am so proud to have been one of the driving forces that brought the program to life – and with it, knowledge and empowerment to young people all over the country.

It is such a joy to know that young people across Australia are learning about their bodies, which will lead to a better understanding of menstrual health, early intervention for those with endo, and more empathy and consideration by teachers and students of people living in pain. It's about time!

The second thing I did after diagnosis was write a comedy cabaret show with my husband, Matt. *Endo The Road* was the first iteration of the show. We did one night only at the 2020 Adelaide Fringe because I thought, *Pfft, who's going to come to this?* We sold out. Endo patients were ready to laugh, cry and join a singing support group where one of their own was telling their story and sharing their experiences. In 2021, we changed the name to *Endo Days,* then wrote original songs, did a longer season featuring a full band (Matt Trainor on guitar and vocals, Sam Jozeps on keyboard, Dylby McCullough on bass and Tina Donaldson on drums – oh and me on vocals, kazoo, jokes, harmonica and questionable burlesque). We've done a lot of shows and it's the best fun I've ever had. It's therapeutic, it's fun, it's educational, it's rude and it validates the feelings of the audience who are there as patients, carers, supporters and even health practitioners. Without comedy and cabaret, I am not sure what would have become of me after all those pregnancy losses and all that heartache.

The third thing I did was write this book, which joins a huge amount of writing about an issue that is ironically underfunded and under-researched.

Although it was first documented on papyrus in 1500BC (seriously!), endometriosis only really started to gain traction as a serious illness in the 1920s when some papers were published on the condition, starting discussion and inspiring more research. Since then, we've moved slowly towards some awareness and recognition of the illness. Social media has been a huge factor in endo patients realising they're not alone and rallying together to keep up the fight for early intervention, better treatment and more research.

The delay in diagnosis time is slowly decreasing with every step we take towards educating ourselves and each other. There is much more awareness now and we are learning so much more about our bodies.

I'm not angry with Dr Ned Kelly, Dr Eye Roll or even Dr iPad anymore. They were all still learning. I am still learning – though they could have been far more sensitive.

I do know, though, that if I'd been better equipped to say what I needed and what I wanted, I could have had treatment earlier. Doctors can't be all things to all people; each patient can afford to learn a little more about their own body and listen to what it's trying to tell them. And doctors, you can definitely afford to listen a little more as well. Let's do this together.

Where to from here: advocating for your body

Patients need to ask questions. Use the resources available, take notes in your appointments, take a friend to your appointment to ask the questions for you in case you get stage-fright. Write your symptoms down so you can say, *This is what I'm feeling. This is what my body is doing. This is what I need.* Ask for a referral to a specialist; seek second or third opinions if you're not comfortable. (But trust that many specialists know their stuff. It's more about finding the specialist that best suits you.) Most importantly, trust yourself. You live in your body and you know it better than anyone. Your health and safety are imperative, so find a healthcare team with whom you feel safe and comfortable.

For each doctor with zero interest in your health condition, there are plenty more who genuinely care. I work on endometriosis and pain with so many health care professionals who are passionate, genuine and dedicated to making a positive difference to people like me. Many are quoted in the following pages. In fact, I probably wouldn't be upright and spritely today without them.

Someday soon, conversation and knowledge about endometriosis and its associated conditions will be as common as those surrounding asthma or diabetes: illnesses that affect a similar number of patients. And when that day comes, when we're all super-knowledgeable about our insides and we can go to a doctor and confidently say, 'I'd like you to refer me to a specialist who can help me with the following symptoms . . .', then we can all find something more pressing to get our knickers in a twist about.

Tips for your GP visit:

1. Take someone with you as an advocate and ally.
2. Write down your questions beforehand and tick them off when you've asked them. Write down the answers.
3. Use a period tracker app and record your symptoms on it so you can show the doctor your data.

4. Research gynaecologists and take the name of the one you want to see to your appointment.

5. Ask for a referral to a gynaecologist of your choice.

6. Use a script if you feel it will give you more confidence.

7. If you aren't happy with the results, make an appointment to see a different doctor. You can often find recommendations for GPs and specialists in online support groups. But remember, everyone has different needs, so their negative experience with a doctor might be an excellent one for you. Don't completely rule out a practitioner based entirely on one person's opinion (but if it's an overwhelming number of people saying that doctor is an exhibition of red flags and alarm bells, steer clear).

Tips for your gynae visit:

1. If your specialist will also be your surgeon, you will need to feel comfortable with them. So if their bedside manner or demeanour doesn't suit you, you can choose to go and see someone else. There is no rule that says you can only see one specialist. It's so important to feel safe.

2. As with your visit to the GP, take someone with you, write down your questions and answers, and show your period tracker data.

3. Write down where your pain is and what it feels like (stabbing, dull, shooting, aching etc) so you can describe it to the gynae.

4. If fertility is a factor for you, try to see a gynaecologist who can help you with that, even if it's down the track, so they can walk with you through your entire journey.

5. Ask about the best treatment plan for your pain, including medications and allied health. If you have allergies or worries about side effects, now's the time to bring them up.

6. If you are uncomfortable about using hormone treatments like the contraceptive pill or Mirena,[6] ask what alternatives they suggest.

7. Ask about costs and private health insurance for appointments and surgeries. Some of the costs can be the surgeon's fee, anaesthetist's fee, hospital excess, and other bills that you might need to budget for, so it's good to be up front about it and have it all laid out for you.

8. Ask if they perform ablation or excision and what the best option for you would be.

9. If your endo is in hard-to-reach places, ask if they will be prepared to bring in another surgeon or whether they will be performing the whole procedure themselves. Some laparoscopic surgeons are happy to operate on the bowel and bladder, while others prefer to have a colorectal surgeon or urologist on board.

10. If you are booking in for surgery and you need to request time off work or school, ask your gynae how long you will need and have them prepare a doctor's certificate for you. (Be aware that your recovery time will depend entirely on what they find and do in your laparoscopy and how your body reacts. So my advice is to overestimate the time you need to recover. If you need less time, bonus! If you need more, at least you've given yourself some leeway.)

11. You can ask how long you might be in hospital for, but it will depend on how your surgery goes and what your doctor finds. Take an overnight bag with loose-fitting pyjamas (nothing tight on the waist – a nightie is best), a comfy change of clothes, a book to read, toothbrush, hairbrush,

---

6 A Mirena is a T-shaped hormonal intrauterine device (IUD) inserted into the uterus, where it slowly releases the hormone progestin. As an aid for endometriosis, the Mirena thins the lining of the uterus and partially suppresses ovulation. It is also used as a contraceptive.

your favourite shampoo, conditioner and bodywash (you'll sometimes feel a bit gross after surgery and want to wash it off you and your favourite smells will really help), and most importantly . . . your phone charger!

12. Ask your surgeon how to prepare for surgery and what to prepare for recovery. Also, ask them for contact details you can use after surgery, for if you are worried or concerned. Everyone's recovery is different and sometimes you need to ask questions like, *why do my incisions look inflamed, is this pain normal?*, or *is this bleeding normal?*

13. Ask to see the photos and report of your surgery at your follow-up appointment. This helps in future surgeries and in planning your long-term treatment. It's also really interesting to learn more about your body and your illness.

2
Endo

a quick, basic introduction

How are you going so far? Shall we just take a moment to revisit the basics? Let's look at endo in a nutshell. This chapter covers the life and times of endo, giving you a potted history and a summary of what it's all about.

What the hell is endometriosis?

Endometriosis is an illness where lining similar to that of the uterus grows on places it shouldn't – like the bladder, bowel, pouch of Douglas (a space or pouch between the rectum and the uterus – don't get me started on a bloke 'discovering' this area and naming it after himself), ovaries and more. It can cause pelvic pain, pain in the legs and back, pain during sex, pain urinating or during bowel movements, severe period pain, ovulation pain, fertility issues, fatigue, low mood and associated conditions.

Different endo patients have different experiences with the illness, which is why it can be difficult to diagnose. Some have extreme, debilitating pain, others have heavy bleeding and fatigue. Some have no symptoms at all and only discover they have the condition if they have fertility issues, a hysterectomy or something unrelated. Some might never know they have it.

The stages of endo are ranked one to four, with one being the least amount of lesions and four being the most. 'Lesion' means abnormality, so an endo lesion is the growth of something (endometriosis) somewhere it shouldn't be.

We now know the severity of your condition doesn't equate to the amount of pain you have. You might have stage-four endo and not much pain or stage-one endo and debilitating pain. It doesn't make sense, but it is what it is. Until more research is conducted into this condition, that's what we know.

So, when folks proudly declare that they have stage-four endo and it's the 'worst case the doctor has ever seen', they might want to consider that the person next to them with stage-one endo might then think their condition is less significant. That might discount that person's struggle and challenges and make them less willing to seek help. We don't want that.

I've told you my story, so you know my endo is stage-four. But my condition is no more important, nor necessarily more severe, than someone with stage-one endo. I am no more deserving of care, support or sympathy than anyone.

How do I know if I have endometriosis?

The most effective way to diagnose endometriosis is via laparoscopic surgery, but there have been some advancements in technology – and work by groups like Aussie research group Imagendo – that might mean advanced MRI (magnetic resonance imaging) scans could become an efficient and accurate diagnostic tool before surgery. These scans could give your surgeon a better idea of where the endo is, so they can remove it and have a good look around for other issues: the scans have already mapped out where the lesions are.

But for now, laparoscopy is the gold standard, and the only way you can be formally diagnosed with endo. Laparoscopy is where a series of incisions are made in the abdomen while you're under anaesthetic and a small telescope is inserted to locate endo lesions. Surgical tools are used to remove the lesions via ablation (burning or cauterising) or excision (cutting the lesion out). It's usually day surgery, with the possibility of an overnight stay, unless your doctor wants you to stay longer.

Remember, excision is the procedure that cuts the whole endo lesion out and ablation burns it off the surface. So, think of it like weeding the garden: if you remove the weed from the surface of the ground without taking up the root, it will look lovely and neat, but the weed may still be growing underneath. If you pull the whole thing out, it is gone and hopefully won't grow back in that same spot again.

What am I meant to do if I've got endo?

Surgery is not a cure for endometriosis. A long-term treatment plan and health care team is required for endo patients to manage their condition. Below are some of the treatments and behaviours that can help manage your endometriosis.

Pelvic pain physiotherapy – helps with muscle spasms, pain with sex, chronic pelvic pain, and other muscular and pain concerns. Your physio will provide you with exercises and stretches that will help loosen those tight muscles in the pelvis that cause the shooting pain up your back and hips, and down your legs. It is crucial for people living with pelvic pain.

Mindfulness and pain psychology – important for wellbeing and central sensitisation. Guided meditations created specifically for pelvic pain are available online or from your pelvic physio. They can be extremely helpful and lovely.

Nutrition and diet – a contributing factor to living well with endo. If you can, avoid a diet high in trans fats, which includes processed foods, fried foods, fast food. Try not to have too much red meat. Cut down on gluten, alcohol and caffeine. Basically, anything that is inflammatory. (I am not good at this. I like consuming all this stuff.)

Have more fibrous foods like fruit, vegetables, legumes, and whole grains, food rich in iron like dark leafy greens, broccoli, beans, fortified grains, nuts, and seeds, foods rich in essential fatty acids like fish (salmon, sardines, herring, trout), walnuts, chia, flax seeds. And you should enjoy plenty of food with antioxidants, like oranges, berries, dark chocolate, spinach, and beetroot. (I can do this bit.)

Exercise – is helpful, even when you don't feel like it. A short walk and some stretches – or just the stretches if that's all you can manage – can help a great deal some days. Swimming is good because it doesn't put pressure or strain on the body's core – pelvis, lower back, hips and stomach – so you don't exacerbate your pain.

Hormonal treatments – like the contraceptive pill, Mirena and Implanon[7] can help by suppressing the growth of endometrial cells and stopping or reducing bleeding, thus reducing the growth of endo lesions. Hormonal treatments don't suit everyone, particularly if you have a sensitivity to hormone fluctuations. It's best to work with your doctor to find the best treatment for you. If you don't like how you feel on a certain treatment, you're well within your rights to change it.

Endep – belongs to a group of medicines called tricyclic anti-depressants (TCAs). It's not a painkiller, but it can help with pain, because it changes the way your nerves receive pain signals from the brain. Endep, which is also called Amitriptyline, can help with issues like pain, overactive bladder or bedwetting, migraine, poor sleep, low mood, and more. It will make you drowsy, though, so make sure you use only as directed and speak to your doctor about whether it's right for you.

---

7   Implanon is a rod that is inserted under the skin in the arm, which slowly releases progestogen to suppress ovulation and aid in contraception. Implanon NXT is the only type of contraceptive implant available in Australia.

Pain medications – can help, but it's important to find one that works for your body and won't be detrimental to your ongoing health, particularly your gut. Anti-inflammatories, especially suppositories can be helpful. Paracetamol can be useful on lower pain days. So can period-specific painkillers that contain mefenamic acid, which are effective because they block the production of the chemicals our bodies make called prostaglandins, which cause pain, swelling and inflammation.

However, opioids, while they take the pain away temporarily, can cause constipation, which will make your pain far worse. Long-term use of opioids can lead to decreased pain tolerance, which can worsen pain. Also, for some people, they can be quite addictive. Opioids have their place, especially for post-surgery and in emergencies, but I reckon if a treatment has the potential to make you worse in the long term than when you started, it's worth avoiding.

Heat packs and tens machines – tight or spasming muscles respond to heat, so wheat bags or heat patches can be helpful. Tens machines are small, battery-operated devices that can be worn on the body, with sticky patches that attach to the skin and give out small, electrical pulses, which can be effective in pain relief.

Hysterectomy – does not cure endometriosis, but some people find some relief once they have their uterus removed, particularly if they also have adenomyosis. This is a huge decision and not one to make in a hurry, so find a doctor you feel safe and comfortable with and explore your options.

The history of endometriosis

The first mention of endometriosis in historical data was in 1500BC, where the Ebers Papyrus (Tebas, Egypt) describes a 'painful disorder of menstruation'. Then in 1690, German physician

Daniel Shroen gave a more detailed description of peritoneal endometriosis in his book, *Disputatio Inauguralis Medica de Ulceribus Ulceri*, ('The Inaugural Medical Book of Ulcers') where he discussed complications associated with the disease, like adhesions and endometriomas.

In the seventeenth and eighteenth centuries, English and European doctors discovered endometriosis during autopsies. They documented facts like endo appearing after menstruation, affecting fertility and causing pelvic pain.

In 1860, Carl von Rokitansky published the first detailed explanation of endo. But it wasn't until 1920, when Albany gynaecologist John Sampson became fascinated with endometriosis in his patients and published papers on the disease and surgical treatments, that things started to move forward for endometriosis patients. Slowly. Very, very slowly.

Now in the 2000s, there is still a seven-year average lag in diagnosis for patients. But now we are talking about it, writing about it – and I'm even singing and joking about it in my cabaret shows.

Thanks to feminism, equal rights movements and the power of social media, we have far more of a voice now than we ever had – and endo patients are using it to get the word out about our struggles and successes.

Co-morbidities and associated conditions

Many people living with endo have associated conditions, which can sometimes delay their endo diagnosis, but are also worth treating independently. These can include, but aren't limited to: bowel issues, bladder problems, mental illness, digestive problems, fatigue, chronic pain, migraines, pelvic inflammatory diseases, rheumatoid arthritis, fibromyalgia, chronic fatigue syndrome and auto-immune disorders. That's a lot!

Having endo doesn't mean you'll get all of these things, but it does mean you need to take care of yourself. And be aware we will be prone to certain things – more than people who are not living with endometriosis and pelvic pain.

I know: there are so many things to think about and it's really frustrating. But you're not alone! You are surrounded by a community of like-minded, similar-bodied, differently abled, chronically iconic people who are here to support you.

Join an online community. Catch up with endo friendos, even if it's just to whinge. Go to any and all information sessions about endo and pelvic pain and keep finding ways to live well. Some days, it can feel impossible. On those days, go back to bed and try again tomorrow when things feel more possible. I don't want to smother you in toxic positivity, because you don't owe anyone anything.

Two solid-gold tips – from my endo pals!

1. My friend Amy says to me, 'if you don't make time for your wellness, you'll be forced to make time for your illness'. That means cancelling plans if they will be detrimental to your health, taking a doona day if you need one, and scheduling things around your cycle if you know you'll be struck out as soon as your period comes.
2. Another mate, Sarah once said to me, 'I have never once regretted saying no to doing something I didn't feel well enough to do, but I have always regretted saying yes.' This means if you know you're not up to something, but you say yes because you think it will benefit everyone else, it ends up benefiting no one. Listen to your body. It knows.

3
Ms Diagnosed

four women, three different backgrounds, one story

Adelia: diagnosis makes a difference

Adelia grew up in Brazil and moved to Australia in 2009 with her partner, Cass. At fourteen years old, she first recognised symptoms of endometriosis. She spent almost thirty years living with the pain until her eventual diagnosis at forty-three. Adelia is friendly, fun and damned tough. She comes across as the life of the party, the leader of the pack – and someone strong as an ox, who would fight to the death for you in the face of injustice. Adelia is great.

'When I was sixteen and in high school, there were times when I had my period and I couldn't go to school. I would spend three days at home,' she says. 'I had lower back pains and I thought it was my spine. I used to pass out because of the pain. I would bleed a lot. I would end up in emergency a lot.

'In Brazil, I went three or four times to a gynaecologist. I had one who did all the tests and then patted me on the shoulder and said, *When you get married, that will sort itself out. That pain you have at the moment will go away when you have kids.*'

Cass and Adelia have been together for more than a decade, and have been through a lot with this illness. Fertility nurse Cass has watched Adelia's illness worsen over time. They both shared with me their frustrations, particularly with the aforementioned specialist. The pair are generous with their time and story, and we sit chatting, sipping on coffee at a busy cafe on Kaurna Land.

'I think he knew she wasn't interested in men, but was still saying, *Get yourself a man and he will fix you up*,' Cass says.

'I told him to stick that up his backside,' Adelia laughs. 'He was telling me as soon as I get a real fuck, it will sort it all out inside. I looked at him and said, *You are such a fucking prick. If I knew you were going to say that to me, I would not have even wasted my time to come and see you.* The door was open when I called him *such a fucking prick* and I made sure that everybody could hear me – and I refused to pay for the consultation.'

Although we spend a good few minutes belly-laughing about Adelia's brash response to her Brazilian doctor, what she's gone through to get a proper diagnosis has put a strain on her life, her fitness, her career as a chef and her relationship with Cass, especially after a neurosurgeon told Adelia the pain was psychosomatic.

'It's hard to watch because there's nothing you can do,' Cass says. 'And I feel really guilty because I know the signs of endo and she's been complaining of pain for a long time. She had a fall about five years ago and it was only after that the pain significantly increased. We had multiple scans on her back and different injections in her hip wondering where this pain was coming from. I did ask for a pelvic ultrasound because I thought maybe it was endometriosis because of all that pain she had when she was a teenager, but the scan came back clear. I thought the only thing was a laparoscopy, but she's terrible with any medications or anaesthetic.

'When the doctor said it was all in her head and we'd done all these things to try to solve the issue, that was hard, because I'm not in her shoes. We'd gone through everything and I thought, what is this? But then there was the guilt when we got the diagnosis. I suspected this ten years ago, but I didn't know enough about it and it's only really in the past twelve months or so that I realise it was all unnecessary pain.'

We all take a moment, because the conversation is clearly upsetting for all of us. It's so hard. The cafe is filled with conversation and the constant thwacking of coffee grounds being emptied and the screeching of the milk frother rival the shrieking of tired children wanting chips and/or to go home. But it seems like we're the only people in the room, because of the bond medical trauma brings to people who have lived it. Cass, a smart, measured woman with the kind of warmth that is immediately disarming, is clearly disheartened by her revelations. Adelia squeezes her hand. 'But we learn,' she says, gently to Cass. 'We learn together.'

The lack of diagnosis slowed Adelia down and put a hold on many of the activities the couple enjoyed sharing together. It was frustrating for Adelia and affected her physical and mental health.

'It's limited what we can do, particularly for about the past five years, because we couldn't ride our bikes,' Cass says.

'And that's something I love to do!' Adelia interjects.

'She didn't want to go swimming at the beach or do anything nice that you'd think would be relaxing,' Cass continues.

'When the doctor said it was in my head, I didn't really want to do anything. The depression came in. I was down for a long time. I would think, *well I'm in pain, but it's in my head,* and with all the people I had seen to try to help me, nobody could. That made me angry and anxious. I was left to suffer.'

'We've been through a lot in our years together,' Cass says. 'And this definitely put a strain on us, but we'd already had so much thrown at us that we've got a great foundation. If we didn't have that . . .'

'You probably would have left me already,' Adelia laughs.

Cass and Adelia are in a strong partnership and despite the enormous challenges endo has thrown at them, they have taken it in their stride. They care for two young children and though life has dealt them some pretty tricky hands, they laugh in the face of adversity and they've got each other's backs. Since her surgery to remove her endometriosis, which happened in her forties, Adelia feels like a new woman. She is exercising again, she's almost completely pain-free, and she's doing all the things she used to love doing. Neither of them can believe the difference a diagnosis can make.

Because, while it's hard to be told you have a chronic, incurable illness, just knowing you weren't making it up, or being over-dramatic, or getting your knickers in a twist – that you have an actual condition that you can begin to manage – makes all the difference.

Claire and Adriana (and me!): diagnosed at 36

Glamourous, charismatic and charming New Zealand-born artistic director and theatre-maker Claire is one of the most energetic, engaging and dynamic people I've met. But her illness is gradually slowing her down, which is frustrating and disheartening for her. She was fourteen years old when she first showed symptoms of endometriosis and pelvic pain and, like me, was diagnosed at thirty-six.

'When I was fourteen, they thought it might be a problem with my hip, then later in my early twenties, they said chronic candida. I had seven years of Implanons – the third one caused me to bleed every day for a year – and during that time, pain and symptoms were controlled,' she says. 'Then the diagnosis was, again, chronic candida and imbalance of pH in the uterus, depression, vulvodynia, appendicitis.'

Adelaide business owner Adriana was also fourteen when she first presented with endo symptoms. Coincidentally, she was also formally diagnosed at thirty-six.

'At fourteen I just thought everyone was putting up with that much pain,' says Adriana, who has had to make many accommodations to make work and home life accessible for her. 'When I was twenty-one, a GP suggested I could have endo and sent me to a specialist who said the only way to check was very invasive. For years I mentioned it to each new GP and they all just nodded and happily let me take Nurofen and codeine to cope. Eventually I went to see an

OB-GYN about something else when I was thirty-six. She sent me for an internal ultrasound and endo was confirmed. I had ovarian endometriosis lesions that were easily seen. I then had surgery and found that I had extensive endo growing right up and across my diaphragm.'

The similarities between mine, Claire's and Adriana's stories are uncanny. Thirty-six seems to be the magic number. Or at least they would be uncanny, were there not so many of us with matching tales of woe.

Claire had her appendix removed in 2017, two years after her endo diagnosis, when two of her then medical team didn't believe that that endo lesions could have returned. They told her it was just her mind telling her she was in pain. After she had two months off work and went through seven hospital stays, her endometriosis lesions were finally discovered and ablated, not excised.

Ablation vs excision

Laparoscopic surgery is currently the gold standard for diagnosing endometriosis (rather than scans or ultrasounds), but one of the big discussions for patients and medical practitioners is whether ablation or excision is the better method for removing endo lesions.

Ablation is where the endometriosis lesions are burned off, destroying the abnormal cells where they appear. Ablation can also be referred to as vaporising, fulguration, coagulation or cauterisation.

Excision involves cutting out the whole the endo lesion. It's better for deeply infiltrated endometriosis, and for sending the lesion off to pathology for diagnosis. Robotic assisted surgery is also becoming more popular, which is where the surgical tools are inserted into the body, then controlled externally by the surgeon.

The chronic illness dance

A diagnosis is certainly a relief, because then you can plan around your illness and treat the symptoms. But there is no cure for endo and surgery doesn't always improve the situation. Planning your world around endometriosis can shake up your whole life, as Claire and Adriana describe.

'I have had to change how I live my life,' Claire says. Before her condition worsened, she used to run long distance and go to the gym every day, but she no longer can, which negatively impacts her mental health. 'I'm physically less able to do things that people take for granted. Some days I can barely walk. If I travel on a plane, the flares are so bad that I frequently end up in wheelchairs. I go out less. I have associated fibromyalgia. The fatigue is debilitating. I feel sadder than I used to. I internalise the way I feel – I think from years of not being heard or believed. I'm trying to work through the emotional and psychological impact of this disease.'

'Endo pain has affected my life more than I can concisely explain,' Adriana relates. 'Like with any chronic pain condition, it affects your ability to work and puts strain on your mental health and your finances. It causes fatigue, and impacts your ability to socialise properly and commit to things the way you would like.'

'I am in some level of pain every day of my life,' Claire agrees. 'I have had to reduce the amount of work I do. I'm trying to find a way to work with endo and adeno, rather than work against it and fight it, because that is exhausting.'

Adeno is adenomyosis, which is a condition where glands and supporting structures of the endometrium are found in the walls of the uterus. It can cause pain and abnormal bleeding, and is similar to endometriosis. But it's harder to diagnose, because a biopsy would need to be taken of the uterus, so it can only really be done after hysterectomy. Some formal scans may show signs of adeno in the muscular layers of the uterus, though. I have adenomyosis and it is so painful. Now that my fertility journey is over, my next step will be a hysterectomy. I hadn't been able to do that until now because I wasn't able to let go of the hope I might have a baby, but now I'm ready. I think.

But Claire is right. The chronic illness dance is exhausting. We spend so long trying to work out what's wrong with us, trying to convince people it's real – and when medical professionals tell us it is psychological, we have to come to terms with that. Then we discover our pain (physical as well as mental) *is* real – and have to deal with whatever that means for us.

The irony is that many years of trying to manage mental health issues that may or may not be there can cause serious mental health issues. I fought like hell to solve a problem that didn't seem to get any better. I was in a constant battle: I'd been told my pain and symptoms were in my head, but nothing I was doing to heal my brain was working. I got to a point where I felt perhaps I wasn't fixable – perhaps, I thought, I should be sectioned.

Each time my body was in pain, I would meditate, do some deep breathing, talk it out, go for a walk and do all the things you're supposed to do when you're feeling sad – even though I didn't feel sad. But the pain was still there, which meant my head wasn't letting me get better, right? So it must be self-sabotage, I thought.

I was my own worst enemy. If I wasn't feeling sad, I would look for something to be sad about because I thought my body was telling me I was sad. I was so angry at myself for not allowing myself to be better. Imagine the self-loathing that comes with that! The broken confidence. The internalised anger. The blame.

The power of self knowledge
Imagine if someone, all those years ago, had validated my concerns that the pain in my body was real, rather than in my head. I could have spent my time managing the physical symptoms and being far more kind to my brain.

Imagine if I had known more about my own menstrual health,

rather than just the basics from a book and a dusty overhead projector taught in Year Eight health by an awkward, baby-faced PE teacher who most of us had a crush on. Imagine if I'd given myself permission to care about myself. And imagine if we were all a little more kind about pain and just believed people who say they are suffering.

I have forgiven myself, but it took a long time. I still revert back to those old habits of second-guessing myself and not seeking help when I need it. My pain is real. The rejection sensitive dysphoria is real. And I am sifting through that. I am a work in progress. But I'm a lot less broken than I was and I'm a lot more kind to myself. And I want you to be nice to yourself too.

4

Managing your Endo

Medical gaslighting

A few years ago, I first heard the term 'medical gaslighting'. Gaslighting is a term derived from the 1938 play-turned-film *Gaslight* by British dramatist Patrick Hamilton. The main character manipulates his wife into thinking she is insane by making her doubt her own thoughts and beliefs and convincing her she is imagining things that were actually happening. The term is now used to describe emotional and psychological abuse where someone repeatedly denies another person's reality in order to dismiss them or invalidate their feelings.

'Medical gaslighting' is a term that has been coined to refer to a patient having their condition, symptoms or concerns dismissed and scoffed at. It's particularly used when patients are told by a medical professional that their physical complaints are psychological. Whether it's through lack of knowledge on the practitioner's side or limited research in the area of concern, it's never okay to dismiss someone if they come to you for help.

I can laugh off many of my experiences of misdiagnosis and chalk them up to a mutual lack of knowledge. But there were some seriously disturbing moments of medical gaslighting in there, like the GP who performed a vigorous, painful, unnecessary and inappropriate internal examination and 'breast examination' (fondling is not an examination) on me when I was twenty-three. I went to him to ask about painful periods. He told me I was imagining the pain and was 'clearly highly strung and mentally ill'. That is gaslighting to make me forget the sexual assault that had just happened.

I have become so used to medical gaslighting and being told there's nothing wrong with me that I won't seek medical help if something *is* wrong with me. For example, I kept working on my laptop while my face swelled up from anaphylaxis, figuring I'd just finish one more task for a client before I took myself to emergency. Looking like a giant botox accident, I finally went to the hospital when my throat started to close over and I was rushed in, hooked up to heart monitors and plied with steroids and antihistamines. I still don't know what the allergy was.

On another occasion, I was bitten by a spider and lost the use of one of my arms for around five hours and didn't go to the hospital because I figured I'd be wasting their time with my drama. I was okay in the end, luckily. Libby 1: Spider 0. Then there was the time I fell over onto my shoulder, which dislocated – so I popped it back in, did nothing about it and it's still sore many years later. And then another time . . . well, you get the point. I don't like to seek medical assistance for fear of gaslighting. Don't be like me.

You've got your diagnosis . . . what next?

Once you find a doctor you want to work with, you can receive a formal diagnosis for endo by laparoscopy, which is just one part of a treatment plan. It's important to note that too many surgeries can cause more problems, due to scar tissue and adhesions (adhesions are bands of scar tissue that sticks organs to other organs). Fun fact: having surgery to have adhesions removed can sometimes cause more adhesions, so chat with your specialist about your options.

Repeat surgeries can also make the body more sensitive and susceptible to pain and that's just counter-intuitive. My hormones tend to go haywire when I've had a surgery, so I am happy with fewer surgeries for my condition. But you do what's best for you under the guidance of a doctor you feel safe with.

Getting an endo diagnosis can be such a relief – but then you've got a stack of homework to do. First things first, though: you need to forgive yourself and make time to grieve. There are a lot of changes ahead and there's a lot of stuff to leave behind. It's a good idea to book in some sessions with a counsellor or psychologist to work through the some of the feelings that might come up, like anger, guilt, frustration – and the realisation that endo will make up a large part of your life.

The first step is to identify your symptoms and work out how you are going to have them treated. Researcher Dr Beck O'Hara is one of my heroes and a founder of EndoZone (a one-stop digital platform built for endo patients and healthcare professionals – by endo patients, researchers, health practitioners and experts). She surveyed a group of Australian people who menstruate aged eighteen and over. Her data revealed that the top five reported symptoms of endometriosis included pelvic pain, fatigue, painful periods, bowel upset (constipation/diarrhoea), and abdominal bloating (endo belly). 'Survey participants reported lower quality of life (both physical and mental) when compared to the Australian general female population,' she says.

Once you've identified your symptoms, you'll want to find your cheer squad, which might include a GP and gynaecologist you like and trust, a pelvic physiotherapist for the pain, a pain specialist, a nutritionist or dietitian, and an acupuncturist. Bonus points if those health practitioners specialise in endo or chronic conditions.

But sometimes it takes a while to find a specialist you gel with and who will make you feel safe and sometimes, you have to sift through a range of experiences until you find the right one.

Maddy's story: medical trauma and cultural insensitivity

Yorta Yorta, Dja Dja Wurrung and Gamilaroi woman Maddy, founder of Yarli Creative, relocated to Melbourne due to a lack of suitable medical support for her undiagnosed, painful condition in Kanny-goopna (Shepparton, Victoria), where she was living. She thought she might have better luck seeking care in the city.

However, when she was admitted to hospital after presenting to emergency with debilitating pain, she was treated appallingly, which heaped trauma onto an already stressful situation.

'I was in so much excruciating pain that I couldn't bend over, I couldn't stand up, I couldn't do anything. I was vomiting. I was on the floor. I couldn't move. I said to my partner, *you need to take me to the hospital now because I don't know what's going on. I'm in so much pain right now and I can't function.* He took me to the hospital and the doctors didn't know what was going on either. There weren't any beds, so I had to stay on a small stretcher until they could find me a bed,' she says.

'My partner left and I was in tears. I didn't want him to leave because I didn't know what was going on. When they finally found me a bed, it was 3 am, and they woke me up and moved me, and then the next day they said, *We're going to get you some ultrasounds.* The guy that took me down to the ultrasound area asked me where I was from and I said, *I'm originally from Shepparton and I've just moved down not long ago.* And he said, *Oh, there's lots of Abos in Shepparton.* And I said, *Excuse me? I'm an Aboriginal person.* He said, *Well, you don't look it.* This was in the hospital setting, and I was feeling really vulnerable.'

After a lonely, sleepless and uncomfortable night in indescribable pain in hospital, Maddy was being wheeled in to have an internal scan by someone who had just thrown a racial slur at her. From there, the experience didn't get any better.

'I went in to the ultrasound, and turned out it was an internal.

This was my first internal ultrasound. I was twenty-one at the time. It was a male doctor, which is culturally inappropriate for us. So, I'm lying there and this doctor's doing my ultrasound. I'm screaming and crying because it was just insanely painful. He had a student doctor in there and she was watching. I was very vulnerable. He then went and got someone else, so I had three people at the other end, and I was crying the whole time because it was just incredibly traumatic. I was in severe pain and they were touching something inside that was really hurting,' she says.

'It turns out I had a cyst rupture, and they were poking at it. That was why I was in such a huge amount of pain and, oh, I can remember it. I feel it. I can remember that vulnerability that I felt.'

While a diagnosis was a relief for Maddy, the trauma she had to go through to get there was unnecessary, unacceptable and needs to change. Maddy and I chat about all of this over Zoom while she nurses her baby Yindi, who is an absolute cutie. She's gurgling, giggling and babbling away while we talk. But the memory of that hospital experience has clearly left its mark on Maddy and she shudders, takes a deep breath, gathers her thoughts and continues.

'As an Aboriginal woman, I see that, especially the healthcare industry, need to understand diversity in our people and understand cultural sensitivities and appropriate ways of looking after patients who are Aboriginal and Torres Strait Islander,' she says.

People presenting to hospital in pain shouldn't have to give a lesson in cultural sensitivity and decency before they receive treatment. It shouldn't be up to them to educate their practitioners in their most vulnerable moments. And above all, racism has no place anywhere or any time. What Maddy went through was grossly unacceptable. She has a right to feel safe and she has a right to treatment without discrimination.

And when she left the hospital, she, like so many of us, was given limited resources to work with.

My first endo steps

When I was diagnosed, I was sent home with no information other than the knowledge it was stage-four endometriois and that I should do IVF, and have a baby, then a hysterectomy. That was far too much for me to take at the time; it was too extreme. I didn't want to do that and I didn't want to have endo.

I spent a bit of time researching on the internet, but my confidence was shot. My response to trying to treat this disease was mixed. I was scared to fix something I'd lived with for so long, because I didn't know what life without pain looked like. And there was a strange sense of not feeling like I deserved to have treatment, as well as heavy denial about having a chronic, incurable condition.

I flicked through Dr Susan Evans' book, *Endometriosis and Pelvic Pain*[8], which was recommended to me by a work colleague with endo. I had a vague knowledge of what I needed to do to manage my endo, but I wasn't doing any of it because I didn't really know where to start. We were trying to focus on fertility so I was completely overwhelmed. But when I started hanging out with other people who also had endo, everything changed. I started to piece together my cheer squad.

(Let's get) pelvic pain physio

A few years after my endo diagnosis, I met Claire. She's the artistic director and theatre-maker we spoke with earlier. After a few wines and a very impressive cheese platter (after which both of us suffered the tummy consequences of too much cheese, but it was worth it), she told me she went to a pelvic pain physio. I thought physios were only for elite athletes and old people, and the only thing I knew about them is that they apparently gave pretty good massages, which release tension and loosen tight muscles. Now, a massage

---

8   Evans, Dr Susan with Bush, Deb, 'Endometriosis and Pelvic Pain', Dr Susan Evans Pty Ltd, Adelaide, 2016

in the pelvis, to me, sounded pretty intimate. Claire was adamant that a pelvic pain physio was the best thing for me, so I just outright quizzed her: 'Claire, isn't that just a finger-bang doctor?'

She laughed. 'It will change your life. You won't regret it. Make an appointment. Now.'

Coincidentally, I had an appointment that day at the hospital to talk about fertility. I was having a bad pain day and I fainted in the waiting room (in my defence, it was a very long wait). My doctor was extremely kind to me and, as I lay embarrassed and dizzy on an examination bed, she gave me prescriptions for things like Endep and Voltaren suppositories, and a referral to a pelvic pain physio.

I'll be honest, I was pretty sceptical. I didn't think there was any way a physio was going to help me. I'd heard Susan Evans talk to endo patients in a session about muscle spasms and pelvic floor tightness, but there was still a big part of me that saw physios as part of the *have you tried yoga?* brigade that would always chime in when I was trying to conceive. I was not convinced.

The *have you tried yoga* brigade (HYTY) are the people who want to offer unsolicited advice they believe will cure you of your incurable condition. They'll suggest pilates for miscarriage, keto for asthma and essential oils for a broken leg. Their toxic positivity is something you don't need in your life. Practise this response for the HYTY: 'Thanks for your suggestion, I'm exploring many good options for my illness at the moment.'

They will then likely say, 'Oh but my cousin had the same thing as you and she went on a juice cleanse and now she's absolutely fine.' Try this response: 'That's great. Unfortunately, I have to leave now because I have something extremely important to do that is top secret and possibly involves moving a dead body, bye!' Or whatever works for you.

I digress.

My endo friendos were all speaking very highly of pelvic physios and the good professor Louise Hull recommended I go. So, having been told by the top tier of people in my life, I was powerless against their wisdom and kindness. I made that appointment.

The pelvic floor is a muscle that supports the organs in the pelvis in people assigned female at birth. It opens and closes the openings of the anus and urethra, maintains bladder and bowel control, contributes to sexual function and helps with orgasm.

We're always told to tighten that pelvic floor, but for people with pelvic pain, that can be the worst thing for us. Pelvic physios help to manage pain. They can work with patients to improve sex, particularly if it's painful or uncomfortable, and they can help with bladder or bowel incontinence.

Your pelvic physio will look at your whole life, your habits and your challenges, and work with you to make better choices to improve your pelvic health. They do an internal examination to pinpoint where your muscle tightness is, but they do this only when you're ready and once they've worked with you to determine your symptoms. A good pelvic physio will send you home with exercises, a program to follow to live and feel better, and will give you hope that you can reduce your pain.

So, I met the physio. I told her my story. She was tough, frank, no bullshit. She told me I had to get fit, be healthier, remove stresses in my life.

She said, 'I know your name. You are involved in the endo schools program.'

I was flattered, tossed my hair a bit, batted my eyelashes, 'Yeah, that's me,' I gushed.

'Well why aren't you taking better care of yourself if you have all of that knowledge at your fingertips?' she asked.

Wow, lady. Brutal. Fair cop, though. We made another appointment, and I went home with some homework to do and some changes to make.

Our next appointment was on a day where I was in agony:

a severe flare-up where I couldn't walk. Matt was at work and couldn't take me to the appointment. He suggested maybe I should cancel, because I was in such a bad way. But I had waited ages for this appointment, and I was quite proud that I'd done some of the homework. I caught an Uber to the hospital (which is about a 20-minute walk from home) and I was in tears as I dragged myself into the car. Painkillers weren't even touching the sides and I was moving like I was chained down with weights. Every step was like lightning shooting up and down my body. It was one of the worst pain flares I've ever had, but like the martyr I am, I pushed through and kept my appointment.

In the consultation room, the physio performed a gentle internal to see where the muscle tightness was and taught me how to breathe through and release the muscle tension. She was not a finger-bang doctor. I take it all back.

She found my problem points and showed me where they were, so I could work on the areas myself. We talked about sex and how to ease any discomfort to make it a more pleasant experience, particularly when trying to conceive. She gave me a plan to get better, and it was realistic and achievable. She could see I was resistant, so she gave me exercises and life changes that I could fit in as part of my normal day.

She asked if I was comfortable with vibrators, because they can act as an internal massager, which releases tension and loosens those muscles. A physician prescribing vibrators, masturbation, healthy eating and gentle exercise? Who wouldn't want to get on board with that? Sure beats yoga! (I'm so sorry, yoga fans. I appreciate and respect that yoga is excellent and helps a lot of people, so please don't downward dog me when you see me next.)

We talked through the changes I'd made and she was so proud of me, which appealed to my need for constant validation. And when I left the appointment, I walked down the hallway feeling great, thinking about how I was going to tell everyone what a great experience it had been – and not a finger-bang doctor at all (stop saying 'finger-bang', Libby. Okay, sorry). In the lift, I reflected on my scepticism and how it had completely changed.

I waved goodbye to the receptionist on my way out and wandered outside into the sunshine, feeling the warmth on my face. It was a gorgeous spring day and the parklands were sprinkled with people sharing lunch out on the grass. I caught my reflection in a building near a crosswalk and noted how bright my face looked. I crossed street after street until I reached my front door. My front door!

I . . . I walked home.

I walked home?

Only two hours earlier, I had to crawl to pick up my shoe because my muscles were spasming so badly I couldn't stand up. I could barely walk – and now I'd walked all the way home. Matt came home later that day and I turned on some music and I danced. I hadn't danced in a while. He was so happy, he cried. So, that's my testimonial, right there. If this sceptic martyr can do it, so can you. Go see a finger-bang doctor (I have got to stop calling them that).

Kylie Rankin: a pelvic pain physio's perspective

Kylie Rankin is a pelvic pain physio (not *my* pelvic pain physio but a good one who is extremely passionate about pelvic and sexual health). She is savvy, charismatic and gentle on approach, and she works damned hard to help someone who was living in pain. She's got your back, and your front, and your insides. Kylie has been in the job for more than twenty years, dealing with every single spectrum of the life cycles of people who menstruate: preadolescents, adolescent, prenatal, postnatal, premenopausal, postmenopausal. She knows her stuff.

'I have dealt with women in pain and I would say probably sixty per cent is pelvic pain,' she says. 'I see people who have gone through from specialist to specialist, seen GPs, been prescribed lots of medication, haven't been believed, weren't being understood and really they'd become desperate . . . and as a result of all their pain, they're extremely guarded. They've got extreme muscle spasms and everything is just tight. And it affects them, because they look well on the outside and society's perception of it is quite dismissive, which is just awful.'

Before she landed in pelvic physio, Kylie wanted to be a sex therapist, which she kind of is now, really. She just does a whole lot more than that as well!

'I have always been interested in helping people, but I wanted to be a sex therapist when I was about fifteen,' she laughs. 'I got into psychology, and I didn't really like it. I deferred and became an aerobics instructor and then someone suggested I become a physio. And I thought *physio, what an amazing field!* I transferred over into physio and I haven't looked back.'

Through her career in pelvic physio, Kylie has helped countless people with their pain conditions. She is passionate about empowering women to enhance their wellbeing.

'Women's health is an area of passion and it wasn't until I had my daughter Lily that I understood the full gamut of being a mother, and the fear and implications of being a woman and having pain,' she says. 'Helping people with their pelvic health is such a privileged position to be in. And I always listen. I think that a lot of specialists just say, *Oh, you know, it's part of being a woman, take some Panadol and deal with it.* So many people come to me and haven't been listened to at all.'

Kylie's approach is a holistic one. She works to give hope and guidance to people living with pain, because she knows many of us have been dismissed and ignored many times before landing on her doorstep. That's why she treats the whole person – because there isn't just one answer to the problem. It's an entire approach.

'You have to be kind to yourself. I like to provide hope that you're not broken, and it's not going to be a forever state you will be in. There's hope and, with the right guidance, you can get benefit and relief from your symptoms of pain,' she says.

Pelvic pain can cause guarding and intrinsic muscular changes and global muscular changes. For example, the abdominal musculature gets tight and guarded, and the diaphragm and breathing is affected, which triggers the pelvic floor that can then be completely turned off or completely turned on or a combination of the two.

'I find out what my clients' goals are and what is important to them and what they want to address, because I don't think it is realistic if you start to target absolutely everything at once. Everyone is varied and different, so I think a clinician needs to develop a rapport and get the patient's trust. And, as a medical specialist, I think what we need to do is just be good listeners. I think women need to be kinder to themselves,' she says.

Kylie is raising the bar with her practical approach, her respect for her patients and her desire to listen to what they have to say about their own bodies. She also educates us about what we should be avoiding and focusing on, knowing we are all different, with diverse goals and issues.

'A lot of women heavily weight train and hit the gym absolutely gangbusters, and it needs to be restorative, not detrimental. Intra-abdominal pressure and severe global tension is not going to be a benefit. You need things that are going to nurture and stretch and give you mental wellbeing. Yoga and pilates are good but find what floats your boat. It's not very helpful to tell you to go and do yoga and pilates if that's absolutely not what you're about. It has to align with the individual. It could be swimming. Exercise helps with your endorphins. It helps with the serotonin levels in the brain. With pain you can get depression and anxiety, so those endorphins help.'

When you go to see a pelvic physio, your goals need to be achievable and realistic. If you're anything like me, you're not going to adhere to a program if it's not achievable. You might even rebel against it. Well, I do, anyway.

Kylie is an excellent example of how a health practitioner can genuinely care and work out a treatment plan that will change your life. Endo is a chronic illness, so there are no cures. But there are treatments and pelvic physio is one of the more effective ones.

So, sign yourself up with a pelvic physio and get your pelvis in order so you can relax the muscles, swing those hips and dance yourself into the next chapter of your life.

5 tips for seeing a pelvic physio:

1. Find one who suits your personality and approach. Do you want gentle and kind? Or do you want a drill sergeant who will hold you accountable?
2. Tell them how you feel. This is crucial. Tell them everything about your condition from concerns about sex to wetting or soiling your pants. They can help.
3. Let them know if you don't want them to do an internal and they will wait until you're comfortable.
4. Be realistic and honest about your goals and what you can and want to achieve.
5. Do the things they ask you to do. I know it's annoying because they give you homework to do, but it has the potential to change your life, so give it a go.

Endometriosis: it's not just the lesions

Associate Professor Susan Evans (my fabulous co-writer of the schools program, and author of the endo book I told you about earlier) also told me about pelvic physio. She told me about lots of other things too: pain, sensitisation, pelvic muscle spasms, Diazepam suppositories (the king of all butt drugs) and all the things that are good and bad for our endo bodies. Basically, stuff you should do to manage pain: physically, mentally and nutritionally. There's so much more about this in her book, *Endometriosis and Period Pain*.

But most importantly, Susan let me in on a lesser-known fact (well, lesser known to me). It's not always the endo that's the problem. Now, I know what you're thinking. You're thinking, 'Shut up, Libby! Don't tell me my endo isn't the problem. Doctors have been telling me for years that this is all in my head and you can't come in here with your fancy book and your good looks, telling me my endo isn't the very issue that I have right here in my extremely painful body!' But hear me out. Or better still, hear Susan out.

'I think everyone, no matter what side of the desk they're on and no matter what their background or their health training, needs to get past the lesions,' she says.

We often hear 'endometriosis lesions' referred to when our illness is discussed. Many people think that the lesions are the main, or only, part of endo, rather than all the surrounding symptoms and associated conditions.

Just a refresher: a lesion is an abnormality. It's tissue, or an organ, that has been damaged by injury or disease. In our case, that disease is the endo. A wound is a lesion. So is a wart, ulcer, or abscess. So what Susan is saying is that there is far more to it than those bits of endo that get removed in surgery. Lots of people think the lesions are the main part of endo, but it's one piece of a whole puzzle. Removing them is only one step of your treatment plan.

'Whenever I did laparoscopy and I saw endometriosis, I did not, in any way, believe that I was seeing the extent of the patient's condition. I always thought I was seeing a common, but non-essential feature of pelvic pain syndrome,' she says. 'In other words, what you see is just part of it. The actual condition we don't understand well enough these days is something that affects the whole body and our whole system. And what you see at laparoscopy is important – good surgery is important; but you can't imagine that the lesions are the whole condition and you can't imagine that removing them will fix everything.'

When I met Susan in late 2017, I told her I'd had my second endo surgery in early 2017 and that I was worried the endometriosis had 'all grown back' because I was in pain and still had symptoms. That's when she let me in on the secret (okay, so it's not a secret, but I felt pretty powerful with this knowledge), that there was much more to endo than that.

She said I needed to see a pelvic pain physio, plan an anti-inflammatory diet combined with stretches to alleviate the pain, and try some anti-inflammatory suppositories. I call them butt drugs (which is not their scientific name, but they are butt drugs, so go with me on this).

Butt drugs are brilliant. They absorb quickly, and because they're localised due to being inserted into the very region where the pain is happening, you can get better pelvic pain relief. They don't suit everyone's needs though, so get advice from your GP. And if they give you the go-ahead, get onto butt drugs and thank me later.

She also told me I should read her book: it wasn't enough for me to just have it on the shelf and expect to learn by osmosis. After our chat, it was clear it wasn't likely that my endo had 'all grown back' at that stage (it did come back, just not that quickly). It was more likely I wasn't managing the rest of my symptoms and was suffering with muscle spasms. I also needed help with an overactive bladder and pelvic floor.

'High-quality surgery is essential,' Susan says. 'But repeat laparoscopy is not doing patients any good. It means that the pain is quite possibly involved in different aspects, things you can't see, and is not getting diagnosed and managed and treated. Repeated surgery can actually worsen pain and worsen the sensitisation that goes with pain and it's risky and it's expensive. Lots of surgery is not necessary.

'The other thing to point out is if you've had surgery for endometriosis, when you go back and look at it later on, it is not going to look like a pristine pelvis. I have a burn on my arm and it's healed. It's several years old now and it doesn't hurt me, but it's never going to look like normal skin.

'When you've had laparoscopic surgery around the pelvis, the skin, the surface of the tissues is never going to look completely normal. The more times people have had surgery, the more it will look a bit different. Don't expect that it's going to look like a perfect pelvis of someone who's never had endo and never had surgery. If you keep going back, you can keep on finding little bits and pieces, but that does not mean that they are the thing causing the current symptoms.'

This blew my mind. I had learned my lesion lesson. I realised there was much more to this than I had initially thought, but to be honest, I realised didn't actually know anything at all. I was sent home after my first laparoscopy with no information, no support, nowhere to turn.

This new knowledge and empowerment helped me with my lobbying for funding and awareness. By 2018, I had joined forces with Susan and PPFA and set about writing an endo schools program together. Susan educated me in all things period pain, endometriosis and the neuroscience behind pain, central sensitisation and nerve pathways. (Just the basics, mind you. We didn't have long!) And I started to do some research of my own, start my treatment plan and find my cheer squad.

But while I was privy to the knowledge of an endo expert, there are countless other patients out there who are seeking answers and not finding them. Or they don't know who to ask or where to go. And many health practitioners themselves need more knowledge and training around pain.

Teaching me about my own health was not a bother for Susan. She generously and happily shared her knowledge. She wanted me to be armed with information and she wanted me to recognise my symptoms and have the tools to treat them. She wants this for all people with endo and pelvic pain. And she wants resources and information to be readily available; for people to have knowledge and be empowered to look after their illness with confidence. And for doctors to be educated, too.

'I would like endo and pelvic pain to be nothing special. I'd like it to be just another area of gynaecology that people understand and that is taught well,' she says.

So how do we do that? We talk about it. We write about it, sing about it, share stories, comfort each other, give advice. We use our village to raise a generation of young people who know how to recognise when their period pain is out of the ordinary and support each other if and when they are in pain or need help. But we also need to talk to the older people who have plenty of experience in dealing with pain. We must make them feel validated and assure them that their pain wasn't in vain: they have survived against adversity and we can learn a lot from them. And we include people of all genders, cultures and backgrounds in the discussion. This disease doesn't discriminate, so nor should we!

And do you know what else we shouldn't do? We shouldn't normalise pain and tell people to *suck it up and deal with it*. We shouldn't be quick to tell people that pain is stress, anxiety or depression, especially if they are reporting physical pain. And we shouldn't exclude people who don't identify as women when they are living in pain. We don't like it when we're dismissed, brushed off and excluded so we shouldn't do it to others. We're better than that.

Socialising with endo

Of course, there are times when we try to manage our illness but the circumstances are out of our control. Like pandemics, for example. But the shit-show that was Covid-19 highlighted many ways I should be taking care of myself. Like avoiding busy places, not feeling bad about cancelling social events, and being comfortable working from home. It also raised some challenges for people that highlighted issues with the health care system that need fixing.

In 2020, when the world shut down due to the coronavirus, we had to adjust to a life indoors and away from each other. Introverts rejoiced about not having to see anyone or feel bad about declining invitations, because there were none to accept in the first place.

Extroverts stampeded straight to the internet and went to Facebook, Instagram, YouTube live and Zoom (a new discovery for many) to get the attention they so desperately needed. I am the latter. I struggled without the noise and energy of people. I always need an audience.

What I didn't struggle with was an empty calendar. Seeing events delete themselves from my diary was divine. I so enjoyed not having to worry about scheduling things in around hormones and periods. I loved the freedom of knowing I wouldn't have to attend an event and smile through the pain. And I was a huge fan of not letting anyone down due to my useless uterus. While often cyclical, endo and its associated conditions can be unpredictable, which means that despite one's best attempts to plan a social and work life, a flare-up of pain, an early or late period, or a painful ovulation will bring on pain, anxiety – and, in some cases, incapacitation.

When I was younger, before my diagnosis, if I had a pain or hormone flare-up, I didn't have a chronic illness to blame it on (despite it being my main problem). I thought it was my annoying head stopping me from doing the things I wanted to do, rather than my annoying uterus. With the stigma around mental health, I didn't want to tell people I couldn't go out because my depression was so bad it was making my abdomen hurt until I was doubled over, vomiting and fainting. So, I lied.

It's important to note, at this point, that I am, in fact, a terrible liar. Awful. The worst. My lies are so detailed and far-fetched, you would probably believe them because nobody would be silly enough to make them up. To avoid going to a family lunch when I was in pain, I lied, telling them that my housemates had locked me in my bedroom accidentally and I was trapped and couldn't come. I lied to friends with stories of my family accidentally locking me out of the house so I couldn't attend their birthday. (The locks were a theme.) I lied to boyfriends, telling them I had to work so I couldn't see them. I lied to bosses at bars, telling them I had explosive diarrhoea so I didn't have to work (no one ever asks further questions when you say that).

But when you've cancelled on people or gone home early or needed to sit down in the corner at parties enough times, you stop being invited. People think you're flaky, even when you're at home in bed hugging a heat bag and wishing you were out with your friends or family. Someone once told me they didn't invite me to their hen's night because, 'You wouldn't have come anyway'. I certainly would have, but I might have left early, because it would've been at a bar or club where there was nowhere to sit. I get too sore from standing for too long. It wrecks me for a whole week. But when I'm unwell with an invisible illness, all people see from the outside is me sending my apologies, or turning up, sitting down and leaving early.

The problem is that when I'm well, I am unstoppable (it's not really a problem, it's freaking awesome). I am dancing till dawn, hogging the karaoke mic with an unacceptable amount of Madonna song choices, making everyone stay out way past their bedtimes – I am the ultimate party gal. And from the outside, it might look like I am just choosing to snub your event to go to someone else's, especially when one day I'll be out of action, and the next I'll be right as rain. But that's not the case.

Something that is really important to note if you have someone with a chronic condition in your life is: try not to give up on them. I know it's annoying and I know they let you down. (Especially if they were going to bring the potato salad and now no one is bringing a potato salad, so what the hell are we going to do about the salad diversity situation?) But it's worth keeping in mind that we don't want to be that way. We would much rather be able-bodied and drinking through a penis straw with you at your hen's night than at home feeling like our womb is about to fall out through our rectum.

In fact, you can even help your endo friend put together a kit for when they have an endo emergency which might mean they are able to manage things better and attend your Tupperware party/ brunch/gender reveal high tea after all. (I'm kidding of course. No one wants to go to your gender reveal Tupperware party high tea.)

Endo emergency supply checklist for if you're home with a pain flare:

1. Have a portable endo first aid kit, with pain killers, heat pack, tens machine, anything else that helps you when you have a flare-up. Keep your GP and specialist's contact details here too. IMPORTANT: you must replenish this kit if you borrow from it, because this is your emergency supply.

2. Queensland endo association QENDO have made endo alert cards that you can keep on your person and show someone if you are in pain and having trouble communicating with someone you've sought help from, like paramedics, neighbours, friends or family members. You can grab one from their website, or make your own card that explains what's happening with you, how they can help and who they should call.

3. See a pain specialist who can help you to plan for your endo emergency. My specialist prescribed me with medication to help with my debilitating migraines, which are linked to endo due to my brain being more sensitive to pain. I also have Diazepam suppositories for emergencies, which are particularly useful for muscle spasms that cause pain so bad I'm unable to walk.

4. Keep some meals in the freezer that can see you through if you're unable to leave the house.

5. Find someone you can trust who would be happy to check in on you or bring you things you need when you're hunkered down and unable to get out.

6. Keep a list of comfort movies and TV shows that you can binge while you're not well. When you're in a pain

flare-up, sometimes the brain fog stops you from making decisions easily, so a list can be useful and will stop you from obsessively scrolling through social media watching everyone else go about their business.

Checklist for if you're going out in pain (because you absolutely cannot miss that wedding/birthday/conference):

1. Keep your endo alert card with you, if you have one.
2. Keep water, snacks and meds on or near you. (I keep stuff in the car.)
3. Don't be afraid to try a mobility aid if you need one. I use a walking stick because it helps me when I have to stand up for significant periods of time and have nothing to lean on. It has changed my life. The folding ones are great because you can pop them in your bag when you're not using them. I have a selection of very cute sticks to complement all occasions.
4. Tell someone you trust that you're not feeling well and brief them on what they can do to help you if you need it.
5. Give yourself a deadline. If the event starts at 7pm, give yourself until 8:30pm and if you make it past that, well done! If you leave at 8:30, then you've done what you set out to do.
6. Arrange a seat in advance or seek out a chair as soon as you arrive. Hospitality staff are usually great at helping if you're not feeling well: they are risk averse and would rather make you comfortable than scrape you/your vomit off the floor later.

Self-care: you don't have to be a warrior every day

Managing your endo is about so much more than prescriptions and appointments. It's also about self-care and prioritising your health. There will be times where you simply cannot do the things you want to do, and that's okay. You don't have to be a fighter every day.

Sometimes, the strongest thing you can do is go back to bed and give yourself a break, so you can get back on your feet to do the things you love again. I don't want to be an endo warrior every day. Some days I want to be an endo slob, or an endo flake. I don't want to battle all the time. Sometimes, I want to give in, be a casualty and try again another day. And that's okay. Cancel those plans. Go back to bed. Get up and try again tomorrow.

Self-care can be about leaning into a life of flat-heeled shoes, comfortable waistlines and venues with soft chairs*. I am getting much better at being honest about my condition and trying to be really clear with people when I accept or decline invitations. I know how disappointing it can be when friends say they are coming to one of my events and then they don't show up. I hate being that person and I don't want to let people down, but unfortunately, my body might have different ideas on the day. I have taken to saying things like, 'If my body cooperates, I'll be there' or 'The event falls at a tricky part of my cycle, but I don't want to let you down, so it's a tentative yes.' Then I am giving myself an out, while still being polite and honest. If you feel comfortable you can try that, or something like: 'Look, I would really love to come, but would you mind making accommodations by ensuring there is someplace for me to sit when I can't stand up any longer?' Besides, couldn't we all get better at making allowances for people and ensuring venues and events are accessible to people of all abilities anyway? It shouldn't be a big ask.

---

*   Just on the chairs thing, I would like to start a campaign to return to comfortable chairs. None of this, 'mismatched, quirky, adorable, '80s classroom shabby chic chair' shit. I want cushions and I want a supportive back. When someone says to me, 'Oh I found this cute little place that does an exquisite oat milk latte and protein ball' all I hear is, 'Come to a place where the chairs will pummel your uterus like a schnitzel.' No thanks. Even though I love an oat milk latte. Count me out. My pelvis hurts just thinking about it.

Back to my point, though. Please keep us on your invitation list. Please don't give up on us. Our condition is painful but being excluded is, too. Give us a chance to come along if and when we are well. We'll show you a great time – and we can all do Madonna karaoke together.

5
Endo and Mental Health

Trigger warnings: *suicide, suicidal ideation, self-harm, body dysmorphia/dysphoria*

Each month, when your period arrives, it solves so many mysteries: why your favourite pants felt tight around the waist, why you ate that entire packet of chocolate biscuits, why you cried at a reality television show about home renovation. And why you have a pimple between your eyebrows and one in the corner next to your nostril, where it's really hard to squeeze.

When you are diagnosed with endometriosis, still more mysteries are solved. Why certain foods can give you sensitivities, what that pain shooting down your legs is, why your period pain is so different to everyone else's. And why it sometimes feels like you're about to get a flu just before your period or during ovulation, because your whole body is aching (it's just your hormones letting you know they're here to mess your shit up for a week or two).

But the best relief that comes with an endo diagnosis is the knowledge that you weren't imagining it. That all those feelings were real and now you can start dealing with the cause. The hunt for answers is over – and a new search begins.

Endo in the news: sharing our stories
One of the great things about being involved in the Australian endo

movement is that I have watched the word start to spread. Celebrities with endo are talking about it, journalists are covering the topic in the news, and politicians are asking questions in parliament about it. There is so much more information available these days that, honestly, if your friends, family or work colleagues don't know what endo is and aren't being understanding about it, I reckon they're being wilfully ignorant. Unless they are living off the grid in a small wooden shack atop a mountain, without access to a phone, internet, or books – in which case, we can cut them some slack.

We now have a National Action Plan for Endometriosis. We've got books being written and published about endo from various perspectives, and in diverse styles. We have cabaret shows, stand-up routines, theatrical pieces, journals, songs – and, importantly, an apology from the man in charge of health in Australia.

In December 2017, the then Australian Federal Health Minister, Greg Hunt, gave an apology to people with endometriosis – which took the edge off my imposter syndrome.

'Let me say something on behalf of all of those in Parliament and all of those who have been responsible for our medical system, I apologise,' he said at an Australian Parliament House Friends of Endometriosis event. 'This condition should have been acknowledged at an earlier time in a more powerful way, and it will never be forgotten again.'[9]

Professor Jason Abbott, gynaecologist, laparoscopic surgeon, farmer (yes, really), former chair of the board of Endometriosis Australia and one of the most fun doctors I've met, reckons Hunt's apology was the sweetest moment for him. It came after years of research, applying for grants and advocating for people with endo: but running into dead ends, because no one was taking it seriously.

'The best thing that I've seen is the recognition of endometriosis and an apology from the Health Minister in Australia to say, oh,

---

9   https://speakola.com/ideas/greg-hunt-endometriosis-national-action-plan-2017?rq=endometriosis

we messed up here because we all thought you were kidding when you said you were in pain,' he tells me. 'This recognition was one of the best moments I've had really in endometriosis. Because we've been saying it forever and been ignored. But it's only ever going to be front and centre whilst the patients jump up and down about it.'

Armed with knowledge and ready for battle

Jumping up and down sounds painful, but we do need to keep shouting about it, and so do our partners, doctors, allied health professionals, parents, teachers, everyone. And we definitely need to arm ourselves with knowledge. This seems unfair, because we already shoulder too much of the burden of this illness. But until this thing is mainstream and 'nothing special' (like Susan says), and until there's more research funding for it, we are the source of power.

'I want my patients to know lots,' Jason says when I ask him what he wants for the countless people who front up to his office daily looking for answers and support. 'I want them to know about their periods, I want them to know about their cycle, and what the limitations are, because I think that too many people expect that everything is solvable and that's absolutely untrue. We still have cancer, we still have diabetes, we still have asthma. And those things have all had trillions of dollars in research. Endometriosis has had, in terms of research, comparatively zero, or lower. We're now starting to see a little bit of spending in the research field, which is great.'

Endometriosis is an unpredictable disease with a range of symptoms that differ for each patient. That's still baffling the experts, but at least a dedicated group of people are working solidly to change that.

'Every time I think we are along a pathway to understanding it and taming it, it trips me up,' Jason says. 'There's just no rhyme nor reason to it. You've only got to see fourteen-year-olds who have stage-four disease rip-roaring through their pelvis and crippled in pain, to know that this is an unjust, unequal, and unfair disease.'

But while things are changing in the endo world for the better, we can't go back and change the past or regain what we've lost. I spent a few years post-diagnosis angry at how I was gaslit, ignored, dismissed, laughed at and treated like a fool. I was angry that mental illness seemed too easy a diagnosis to throw on me. (And at the same time, there's nowhere near enough focus on mental health services.) I was angry that I had an incurable, invisible illness and that even though I am now diagnosed, I still seem to attract eye rolls and dismissive doctors.

The lack of awareness, support and resources for endo patients can have seriously harmful effects, as Jason knows all too well.

'Having people understand this disease can be deadly is something we must continue to note. Because if all it is, is just a bit of period pain, then women shouldn't be killing themselves. I've had a number of women in their twenties take their own lives because of the disease and that is not okay. It's not okay.' Jason stops to take a breath. It's very clear this weighs heavily upon him. He's frustrated, he's worried and he's hurting for his patients and others like them.

'We need to continue to change the dialogue of it just being about periods and pain, and change the whole taboo that goes with menstruation. It is still unbelievably sexist. We need to accept that and understand and recognise that it's only by supporting women that everything gets better. Everything. And if we can't do that with women's health, then we're lost.'

Giving hope and providing support

Jess Taylor is one of the most impressive women I know. So young, yet so driven to make positive change. She's strong, no-nonsense, innovative and gets shit done. She's also funny and generous and she has dedicated her life to supporting people with endo, mostly in a voluntary capacity – all while living with the disease herself. She is president of QENDO and like Jason, she has seen the darker side of the illness, through things like the organisation's 24/7 phone support line, which was set up to help endo patients with questions and issues they couldn't find help for elsewhere.

'The worst-case scenarios I've come across are people who have been on the line thinking they don't have any choices in their life, and they're going to end it. And I get it. I've actually also been there, when I was told we might not be able to have a child and I thought, *What is the point? Honestly, what is the point?* And if someone's got to that level, how much has the system completely failed that person?' she says.

'The other side of that is the hopeless. Where they don't know what to do next, they're not considering ending their life, but they literally don't know what to do next. They don't have hope, they don't have anything, they're numb. So that's a very real moment that's often not talked about.'

The thing with this illness is that there's a new strategy, treatment or decision needing to be addressed at every turn. There's a new challenge being thrown at us and a new barrier to try to climb over. That might be getting your pain under control and then realising you now have to plan for future fertility options. Or maybe you're like me and have discovered hormone treatments don't agree with you due to their causing severe mood swings and depression – so how do you keep the lesions at bay? Or maybe it's trying to navigate your relationship and social life. It just seems like we need to be hypervigilant all the time, which is physically and mentally exhausting.

Early diagnosis and knowledge: Chloe, Teagan and Jorja

There are so many things I wish I knew when I was a teenager and in my twenties. So many things that might have changed my life. I always felt like a failure because I just couldn't get well. I am never not tired and for a long time, I just couldn't fix what was wrong with me. I still can't fix it for the most part, but at least now I know why I can't. That lets me go a little easier on myself. When I see people diagnosed with endo at an early age, I'm happy for them because they have knowledge – and knowledge is power. (Though I'm sorry, of course, they now have this tricky disease to navigate.)

Chloe (nineteen) is strong-willed, motivated and studying to be a nurse. She was diagnosed at seventeen after presenting with symptoms from puberty (at around thirteen years old). She had to push doctors to get a diagnostic laparoscopy: they were reluctant to operate on a young person and were convinced her pain was psychological. But she won the battle and can now plan for her future with endo.

'Before I was diagnosed, my doctor told me I had psychosomatic tendencies, so getting a diagnosis was such a relief,' she says. 'I've been able to manage issues which would have snowballed into bigger issues if I was diagnosed later. I have a low egg count and a lot of scarring, so knowing this, my team can be proactive and freeze eggs while I'm young,' she says.

From the age of thirteen, Teagan, who is now studying to be a teacher, suffered intense pain that was accompanied by vomiting, fainting, and hot flushes, which meant she missed school and was living with poor mental health.

'After PPEP Talk® came to my school in Year 10, and informed us about endometriosis and period pain I thought, *Wow, I experience all of these things and more.* I remember putting my hand up and saying I suffer really bad pain for about three days prior to actually starting my period and the lady looked at me and recommended I see a gynaecologist or my local GP. That day, I told Mum, *I believe I have endometriosis,*' she says.

'It was extremely hard to find a gynae who was willing to take on a fifteen-year-old. So after many failed calls, we finally found a gynaecologist and I underwent my laparoscopic surgery in 2019. I was sixteen. I was scared, but looking forward to finding a reason for all my pain.'

After three years of feeling like the pain was in her head, Teagan received her endo diagnosis, with the added extra of a cyst the size of a tennis ball, which was removed during her diagnostic laparoscopy, along with the endo. Having an early diagnosis means Teagan can practise self-care and try to live well with endo.

'I see a pelvic floor physio once every two weeks who helps me to loosen the muscles and find strategies and stretches to do when I am having an endo flare. My mental health has just as much of an impact on my endo as eating healthy and drinking water does. I know my body quite well, and I know that when I am stressed, I tense up, causing my endo pain to be significantly worse. My boyfriend, family and I try to minimise stress as much as possible,' she says.

'By being diagnosed at sixteen, I can confidently say I know my body inside and out, I know all my triggers, I know what foods hurt my tummy, I know what stretches help. I have a Mirena so the spread of endo has decreased massively, which might not have been the case if I'd been diagnosed later.'

I often think about what life might have been like had I known I wasn't a hypochondriac, drama queen or troubled teen. I wish my family had known so they could have understood that I wasn't just being a flake, and I wish I could have communicated better with them. I wish my mother had been told by her mother that debilitating pain isn't normal because then we might not have all pushed through 10/10 pain that would send able-bodied people straight to hospital.

Jorja (sixteen) was diagnosed via laparoscopy when she was fourteen. She is also vision impaired. I met Jorja when she came to my cabaret show, *Endo Days* (twice) and I have to say, this kid is going to change the world. As soon as she was diagnosed, Jorja swotted up on all things endo and taught herself what she needed to do to survive. Then she turned her attention to the endo community and shared what she'd learned with them. She is always jumping in to guide and support people on the online support platforms and she shares her candid commentary on her Instagram page, @endo.jorja.

This young person who is living with the challenges of a chronic illness as well as vision impairment is consistently generous with her time, knowledge and stories. But she's had such a difficult journey so far. I truly hope science can advance fast enough to make sure she has a magnificent, pain-free adult life.

'I started having bowel issues at the age of ten and had chronic constipation and unexplained stomach pain that was put down to anxiety. I started my period at twelve and that's when I started having extreme period pain for up to four days of my period,' she says. 'I had to either take days off or get picked up from school early because I would be crying on the toilet passing clots.

'When I was thirteen, my first ovarian cyst burst. At the time I had no clue what it was and I was probably in the worst pain of my life. My mum thought it was just the constipation, so I just had Panadol and stayed in bed until I could sleep. I eventually went to my doctor because I was still having horrible, acute pain and they found a cyst on my left ovary. Then, after months of trying to figure out what was happening, a GP mentioned endometriosis. I had never heard of it before and no one in my family had either, but the symptoms sounded like they fit. I went on the hunt to find a gynaecologist who could help.'

Due to her young age, some gynaecologists were reluctant to perform laparoscopic surgery, and others were convinced it was nothing more sinister than the occasional painful period, but after a few false starts, she found a doctor keen to work with her.

'Eventually, after a year of chronic pain and trying unsuccessfully to stop my periods with the pill, a gynaecologist who was also an excision surgeon agreed to do a lap. I was diagnosed with stage-one endometriosis and it was such a relief, and also a bit terrifying.

'I ended up having to drop out of school which wasn't ideal, but I was already missing so many days that there wasn't much point. I started online school, which had its own challenges, being vision impaired, but it helped take a lot of the stress off me and gave me lots of time to rest if I was in pain, and the best bit is that I could do my schoolwork in my PJs!'

Jorja's mother is super supportive and has been a tower of strength for her. I'm always moved when I see parents and their endo children banding together to fight the disease, especially now there's more information to share.

My sister Kathryn was recently diagnosed with endometriosis, which we long suspected. Our mum also had the same pain, but we just didn't know about it at the time. It's only decades later that we're learning. At least now I have the knowledge to teach my step daughters, Niamh and Keeley, about managing period pain, and Kathryn can talk to her boys, Kane and Jake, about it.

My mum was only doing the best with what she knew. She had taught herself how to live with the pain and that's what she passed on to us. It's an excellent skill to have and it's served me well throughout my life. But I tell you what, I'm glad I have permission to give in to the pain now. I am glad I have a name for it so I can throw my hands in the air, bow down to the flare and call it a day.

It's great having knowledge about this stuff so I can be nicer to myself. But one of the other great things about seeking knowledge about health stuff is that you meet interesting and exciting people who teach you even more things you didn't know you needed to know about yourself.

A gynae with endo: Dr Sarah Van Der Wal's story

Dr Sarah Van Der Wal is a gynaecologist, obstetrician and person living with endo who lives in Bendigo (located on the traditional lands of the Dja Dja Wurrung and the Taungurung Peoples of the Kulin Nation), and works both there and Echuca.

Sarah is funny, passionate, and damned clever. We have never met in real life, but I appreciate our online friendship, which we found while I was seeking information for this book. Since then, I have learned a little about what it's like to be a queer, non-binary person with endo living in a rural location and working as a gynaecologist.

Sarah told me a lot about their experiences, but also told me they want people to know they should not use soap on their vulva because it can lead to chronic itch. (This is a fun fact and nothing to do with endo or what we're going to talk about next, but I think it's important to note. Use a soap-free body wash or just a face washer and water if you have to, but no soap.) Okay, that's out of the way, let's get back to talking about intergenerational pain trauma.

'I wish my mother had known it wasn't normal,' Sarah says. 'My mother was never diagnosed with endometriosis, but it is twenty-five per cent familial, and there's a strong suspicion that she thought my condition was normal, because it's what she had. I wish I'd known back then to be able to say, actually, debilitating pain is abnormal, and I want someone to do something about this. Because then I might not have inoperable stage-four endo now. Maybe something could have been done, back in the day. It has had an impact on my fertility and it's had an impact on my mental health.'

After unsuccessful attempts with IVF and a toll on their well-being, Sarah and their partner Carla decided Carla would carry their two children. As a patient and a doctor, endo has had a profound impact on Sarah's life – and has made them more in tune with their patients' needs.

'It's completely changed how I deal with talking to people about endo; how I deal with counselling people. I'm very quick to offer a diagnostic procedure, because I think that far too many people are just left not knowing. It's a chronic health condition that's essentially untreatable. You can mitigate symptoms, you can mitigate it with some surgery, but it's going to come back. It's incurable, untreatable, and has a massive effect on people's lives.'

Once diagnosed, Sarah says it's crucial to talk through what that means for the patient.

'It's a grief thing when you're diagnosed with something incurable.

And I think that what happens to a lot of people is they're told, *Oh, yeah, your pain's caused by endo. We'll take you to theatre and we'll cut it out, and it'll be fine.* And it doesn't work like that. People do much better when given realistic – not pessimistic, but a realistic – appraisal that it is chronic' Sarah says.

'Sometimes I disclose my own endometriosis to say, *I actually do understand what you're going through and I'm not just telling you this as part of the medical establishment that has completely ignored your pain for ten years. I'm not dismissing you. It's shit, it's terrible, but I'm here to keep working with you to try and get you to the best we possibly can.*'

The mental load of working through a diagnosis can be a heavy burden for most of us, but it can be even heavier for some people who were assigned female at birth (AFAB) but do not identify as women. These include but are not limited to people who identify as male, transgender, gender neutral, non-binary, A-gender, pangender, genderfluid, genderqueer – or all, none or a combination of these. Some people suffer gender dysphoria, which is the discomfort or distress of a person's body not aligning with their gender identity. They might also suffer body dysmorphic disorder (BDD), a mental illness characterised by a person's fixation or worry about their appearance.

As a doctor who not only has endo but also identifies as non-binary, Sarah says they have become more aware of providing individualised care.

'It makes me help the person in front of me instead of treating people as a homogenous group. I'm more conscious of people's pronouns and identity, and making sure I'm creating the safest space possible for everyone,' Sarah says.

'Treating everyone like they may have had to negotiate a hostile medical system and making sure you're not part of it makes you a better doctor. And being non-binary helps me remember that. I have amazing cisgendered colleagues who do the same; it's not a prerequisite, but it is a constant reminder.'

Not all women have a uterus and not all people with a uterus are women

When I was visiting schools for PPEP Talk®, I spoke with a number of non-binary folks, gender non-conforming people, and AFAB people who identify as male. Some of these people still have a uterus, so the information we were providing is extremely important to them. Because we understood about gender dysphoria and being inclusive, we were very careful about using non-gendered language.

It was really driven home to me when I was a teacher and I was presenting a lecture to an entire year level. I carelessly said, 'Lady at the back, what do you think?' and the student said, in earnest, 'I'm a man'. I apologised hurriedly and clumsily and then approached the young person at the end and apologised again. He said, 'It's okay, but when people call me a lady, I want to kill myself.' My stomach fell. I felt awful. But definitely not worse than the person I had misgendered.

Never, ever again have I used gendered language when addressing groups of people and I am conscious of using the correct pronouns for people. I am still learning and I don't always get it right, but if it saves someone's life, it's worth using non-gendered language. It doesn't hurt me to do it, but not doing it can cause more hurt than I ever imagined.

That's why it's so important to use non-gendered language in online support groups as well. This disease can be lonely, isolating and at times depressing. If you're looking for help but all the help is labelled using language that is traumatic or takes away your autonomy, that's awful. I don't want people to feel worse than they already do – so if I just make a few little accommodations, it can make a huge difference to someone I may not know, but for whom this is a very big deal.

Jamila is twenty-seven, non-binary, an ambulant endo patient. They do not mince words when it comes to their feelings about misgendering.

'I would rather someone fucking punch me in the face than misgender me. That would hurt less. Misgendering is really violent and it's not just saying the wrong word for someone. It's about not seeing that person for who they are. It's alienating, and painful, and frustrating. And it's removing your autonomy when you're already in a situation where you're lacking a lot of independence,' Jamila says.

And seeking treatment in 'women's health' can be problematic, particularly when there's a long way to go in making non-gendered language the norm.

I met Lore in a Facebook group focused on endo and inclusivity and they were candid and generous with me about their difficult journey around menstrual health. Lore hated everything about puberty because they do not identify as female and they were extremely dysphoric. They have since had a hysterectomy after coming out as a trans, non-binary person. Lore and I met via Zoom: I was in Adelaide (Kaurna Land) and they were in Naarm/Melbourne (the lands of the Bunurong Boon Wurrung and Wurundjeri Woi Wurrung people of the Eastern Kulin Nation).

'I didn't know it was dysphoria until I figured that I was trans. I am asexual (ace), and when I was twenty-three, I had a sexual assault, so I had trauma around that area as well. So, that made everything more intense,' Lore says. 'I was disassociating from any secondary sexual characteristics that didn't match my brain. I couldn't look at myself in the shower or stand the idea of someone else looking at me, which would just confirm my body was what I didn't want it to be. It was just completely overwhelming. And even now, I've had top surgery for my chest, which is great. But if I go to a gynaecologist, I find it hard to deal with my body or have anyone else looking at it.'

Due to the dysphoria and trauma associated with Lore's experiences, misgendering them can have a profound effect, like the time a nurse rubbed pronouns off the whiteboard above the bed when Lore came out of surgery because she didn't think it was necessary to have them there for Lore.

'Whenever I'm trying to find information relevant to me about endo or ASD [autism spectrum disorder], it's always super gendered, which is like another arrow, another barb. Sometimes it's the straw that breaks the camel's back, and I'm done with life for the day. Other times, I can clench my teeth and try to brush it off. Tiny little micro aggressions add up when it's in every facet of your life,' Lore says.

But it's not just the language that can ruin someone's day. The transition medication for Lore, who is a sex-repulsed asexual person, gave them an increased sex drive, which was confronting and distressing.

'I was on low dose T [testosterone] for six months prior to my hysterectomy, but I have kept my ovaries because I am non-binary and still figuring out how I want to present. And my libido was annoying as an ace person because I don't want to be thinking about something I don't want to do anything about,' Lore says.

I met Lewis in the same inclusive, online endo support group, Inclusive Support For Endo and Other Pelvic Pain Conditions Australia, and we talked for hours. I learned so much from both Lore and Lewis and I am grateful they took time to educate me about things that are unfamiliar to me, but make up so much of their lives. It is, of course, not their responsibility to do this and I am aware of the toll these conversations would have had on them. They both opened my eyes to so much that I didn't know, but can now be more sensitive to. Lore and Lewis both wanted people to understand what they're going through. But gosh, it must be exhausting for them having to do that all the time, particularly in a health setting.

Like Lore, Lewis is living in Naarm (Melbourne). We went off on many tangents during our conversation and every time we went to end the Zoom call, we would find something new to talk about.

Lewis, who is non-binary and an endo patient, tells me that some of the biggest gendering confusion happened when they were at the

Royal Women's Hospital because people often confused them with being a visitor rather than a patient, because of their masculine appearance.

'Once, someone presumed I was as a staff member. I've been at that hospital quite a few times, but I still feel so uncomfortable. People don't quite know how to read me and often presume I'm someone's partner, rather than a patient. I seem to usually get read more as a man, which is great,' Lewis says, earnestly.

'I must say at least the receptionist for my physio has been wonderful, as has the physio themselves. The receptionist edits the reminder letters for appointments, takes out the word "woman" and puts "person".'

I am one of the admins for the South Australian based online support group, Endo Support SA. There, the topic of gendered language comes up sometimes. But a vast majority of people are respectful and follow a rule we made about mandatory inclusive language. We ask people to use language and greetings that include our trans and non-binary friends. Rather than, *Hi sisters, Hey ladies!* or *Hi girls,* we prefer people to use greetings like, *Hi friends, Hey everyone,* or *Hi folks.* Sometimes people who identify as female don't understand the huge effect those words can have on someone who is already vulnerable, looking for support, experiencing dysphoria and feeling excluded from what should be a safe space.

Put it this way: think about a word that really grinds your gears and then imagine people are saying it to you all the time, often in your safest places and sometimes knowing full well it will upset and exclude you. For me, it's people, especially cis (short for 'cisgender', and meaning your gender is the one you were assigned at birth) men, calling me *love, dear* or *sweetheart.* I find it condescending and infuriating, and if it were happening every day, even if people have been told to stop, it would amplify my hatred of it and make it even worse.

'I have dysphoria about having a uterus and having ovaries,' Lewis says. 'I did the egg retrieval process and I had a very bad time with those hormones. I was really sick, and when I had to talk to people about it in a place that's mainly for cis women who want to have kids, I really felt I didn't belong there. It was awful. I felt quite ill going through the process because I thought, *I don't want this part of me (my uterus), but I'm doing this anyway just in case I get a hysterectomy and then in a few years I think, what have I done, maybe I do want children?* But I get such dysmorphia about anything pregnancy related.'

The world is constantly changing and with it, we have to as well. Sometimes that can be uncomfortable, but it if it saves a life, I reckon it's worth it. And the best bit about the world evolving is that endo patients are getting smarter and stronger – with more knowledge, feeling more empowered and more willing to share stories and resources.

The endo revolution: we ride at dawn

Jess from QENDO reckons patients will rise up. Not in a rebellion sort of way, because we are tired and crampy and don't have the energy for a physical confrontation or frontline street-fighting. (Although, I'm happy to gesticulate wildly from my recliner lounge when the revolution begins.) But Jess is talking more about a medical enlightenment for patients.

'Patients and advocates are going to become clever,' she says. 'They're going to become even smarter than they already are, and the medical field needs to get on board with that. We no longer have a community of people who are just going to accept whatever is said. We're going to see generations coming through who will question things. And doctors only have fifteen minutes of their patient's day, so they need to work out how they are going to listen and communicate better.'

That fifteen minutes in the workday of a GP can mean the difference between being directed towards a specialist for further investigation, or another fifteen years of wondering what's wrong and living with an undiagnosed illness. I respect that doctors can't know everything. That would be impossible. But it's unfortunate that I visited *countless* doctors who used that fifteen minutes to dig their heels in and dispute what I was telling them. I may not have had all my information in order, and I certainly wouldn't have used the correct words, but didn't I at least deserve a chance to be heard?

I'm learning to let go of all that, because life is too short and my mental health is more important. I read somewhere once that anger and resentment is like holding onto a hot coal waiting to throw it at someone. I had been holding on to those burning coals long enough and the only person it was hurting was me, so it's time to move on.

That said, I have now learned when to get angry and stay angry if it means taking action to improve things for the greater good, like fighting for endo awareness and education. I know this type of directed fury comes with age, but it also comes with tragedy. Someone once told me that 'ultra-independence is a trauma response'. Having gone through eleven pregnancy losses, an armed hold-up and countless interactions with dodgy men – on top of medical gaslighting and misdiagnoses – I don't like to rely on anyone. I like to do things myself. And up until recently, it was a case of: *if I can't do it myself, I simply don't do it.*

But I've been forced to change that. Forced to start delegating, trusting, relying, collaborating – all words that once scared me, but now (sometimes) make me feel safe. I am working to create important projects that make me happy and help others. I'm being honest with people about what I can and can't do, and I'm trying not to feel like a failure if I can't do things.

Self-talk: be kind to yourself

Most importantly, I've learned about self-talk to improve my mental health. Self-talk is that little voice in your head: you know the one. It's your internal dialogue when you're sad, unhappy, excited or winning. It commentates your day. Self-talk is different to real talk, but it probably shouldn't be.

Think about how you talk to your friends, family or workmates when they're down, when they're angry, when they're falling apart, when they succeed or when they're on the right track. Then think about how you talk to yourself when you're sad, made a mistake or completed something important. Compare the two. Are they the same? Good for you! Keep up the good work! Are they vastly different? Thought so. Why is that? Why do we talk to ourselves like that?

If someone finishes something important, I'll say *Well done!* If I finish something important, I think *Hmmm should probably have finished that sooner and it's probably not very good.* But think about this: if your friend came to you and said, *Hey, I think I really messed this thing up at work and I am pretty sure I'm going to get fired, even though it probably wasn't that a big deal but I'm really worried,* would you say, *Of course you're going to get fired! You messed that up so badly and everyone is talking about it? Also, everyone hates you.* No, you wouldn't say that to your friend! (I really, truly hope you wouldn't.) So why do we talk that way to ourselves?

Imagine this scenario:

Libby 1: Oh hey, Libby. I'm feeling a bit down at the moment, because I'm really tired and my period is coming. I want to tell my friend that I can't come to their party on the weekend because it's at a club and I know there won't be any seats there and I won't be able to stand up all night.

Libby 2: Oh yeah, she's gonna hate your guts. She'll definitely dump you as a friend and tell everyone how shitty and unreliable you are.

Libby 1: Yeah you're right. I'll probably end up going anyway and pretending to be okay, but I'll end up in debilitating pain for the rest of the week and have to take time off work.

Libby 2: Oooh, your boss is going to be so mad at you! I bet you get fired.

Libby 1: I don't want to get fired! Maybe I'll just say I can't go to the party then!

Libby 2: Yeah 'cept then everyone will hate you, so choose between no job and no friends, loser.

End scene.

Maybe if you changed that into a conversation where you behave as if you're talking to a friend, it will be more like this:

Libby 1: Oh hey, Libby 2. I'm feeling a bit down at the moment, because I'm really tired and my period is coming. I want to tell my friend that I can't come to their party on the weekend because it's at a club and I know there won't be any seats there and I won't be able to stand up all night.

Libby 2: That's a good idea. You need to look after yourself so you can get through the week. She'll understand. Perhaps you could offer to take her out somewhere special to make up for it when you're feeling better.

Libby 1: But what if she gets really mad with me?

Libby 2: Well, you haven't got a problem until you've got a problem, but if she gets mad, maybe it's time you distanced yourself from someone who doesn't understand your condition and revisit the friendship when you're feeling stronger.

Libby 1: That's great advice. Thanks, Libby 2.

Much better!

Hormones, problematic PMS and endo

Despite making changes and improvements in my life to allow for better mental health, I can't control what my hormones do to my brain (they pretty much break my brain). I have never been able to take the Pill or any other hormone treatments to treat my endo, because the change in hormones affects me too much. I'd tried to take the Pill plenty of times for contraception, but I would just feel so sad, agitated and hopeless. When I stopped taking it, I would bounce back to normal, but my PMS (premenstrual syndrome) has always been terrible.

Since being diagnosed with endo, I've learned hormone treatments can help keep the lesions (thus the pain) at bay because they suppress the cycle. But the thought of putting hormones on top of my already wacky hormones has always been an unwelcome suggestion. Many people have success with the Mirena and other IUCDs (intrauterine contraceptive devices) but for some, it makes them feel worse. That's why it's good to find a treatment that works for you, in collaboration with a doctor you feel comfortable with.

I had visited many doctors to talk about my pain and my problematic PMS, but the diagnosis was always 'depression, anxiety, stress' and the treatment was the Pill or antidepressants, both of which made me feel worse. I spoke to GPs about my PMS, but they would always put me on the Pill and I ended up on a big, scary hormone merry-go-round that was no fun for anyone.

I tried to talk to a doctor about my wild hormones and mood swings when I was in my early twenties and married to my first husband David (a sweet, sensible, introverted man who was the very opposite of me and my chaos and noise, which clashed hard with his zen, ensuring the marriage ended very quickly). I wanted a cure for the absolute turmoil I was going through just before my period. 'I'm a monster!' I told the doctor, sobbing. 'I'm just not myself! I am irrational, paranoid, anxious, ragey. I make kneejerk decisions that are always the wrong ones. I'm never violent or angry, just quick to frustration, easily agitated and will swing between fury and sadness and then over to extreme arousal in a single minute.' The doctor said, 'Yes, you have bipolar and needed to be medicated to save other people from you.'

'But I'm only like this before my period!' I argued, knowing full well that as soon as my period came, a wave of calm would wash over me and I would be back to my chilled self for three weeks – making bad decisions because I wanted to, not because my hormones were telling me to.

'No,' he said. 'The agitated person is your real self. The calm you have from your period is actually the fluctuation of your hormones affecting your mood. The real monster is you.' And then he chuckled and wrote me a script for another antidepressant.

I took home his prescription and added it to the pile I would never end up filling. I'm not anti-antidepressants. I think they are marvellous if they work for you. I just never had any luck. I was prescribed them for what I'd later discover was endometriosis and adenomyosis, as well as PMDD. So they just made me feel like I was walking through treacle with a brain made of marshmallow, nauseated every day and fighting insomnia – without taking away any of my other symptoms. Then I'd feel like a failure because they weren't working, so I'd stop taking them, go back to the doctor, get another unfilled prescription and the cycle would continue.

Premenstrual dysphoric disorder (PMDD)

I was forty when I discovered there is such a thing as premenstrual dysphoric disorder (PMDD). It's like premenstrual syndrome (best known as PMS) but far more severe. It's PMS on crack. PMS causes irritable mood, but doesn't tend to interrupt your daily routine. PMDD can absolutely derail your whole week. Symptoms include (but are definitely not limited to) fatigue, paranoia, depression, suicide ideations, anxiety, short temper, decreased libido and heightened sensitivity. I'll let you know at this point that there are doctors who don't believe PMDD is a thing. I am not a doctor but I live in my body and I know what it does as soon as there's a hormone fluctuation, because my whole world turns upside down.

PMDD usually happens ten days before a period starts. In my case, I can set my watch by it. As soon as I start to feel that swell of sad/frustration/angst, I'll look at my period-tracker app and it will say, *ten days to go*. Every time. Without fail. My best mate Amy, who also has endo, was the one who 'diagnosed' me. Amy isn't a doctor, but I felt like she was a goddamned scientific genius when she told me about this PMDD thing.

'Do you feel angry for no reason, frustrated with everything and you want to kill yourself even though you don't really want to kill yourself but it seems like the only logical solution?' she asked.

YES.

'Do you feel like you're the worst person in the entire world and probably the cause of all world wars and also poverty, but as soon as your period comes you realise that's silly because you're only responsible for your own ridiculous choices?'

YES.

'You've got PMDD.'

OH. MY. GOD.

'Stop shouting, I am very hormonal.'

What a game-changer! I finally had a name for the thing that made me feel like I was Hannibal Lecter/Darth Vader/Ursula the Sea Witch (choose your own fictional villain) for a few days – before I just got on with my life like nothing had happened, knowing I wasn't inadvertently responsible for everyone's unhappiness.

A doctor friend heard me talk about PMDD, rolled her eyes and said, 'yes, it's a mood disorder' accentuating the word 'moooood' so it sounded more annoying, silly and eye-rolly. Yes, it is a disorder that affects moods, but let's not dismiss it – or any disorder that affects your mental health. Having PMDD is like being allergic to your own hormones. It's an adverse reaction to the hormone changes in the luteal phase of your cycle. And as soon as the hormones shift, the change can send the person into meltdown.

Catching my sleeve on a door handle will make me think I am a personal failure and that nothing I do will ever be any good. Dropping my keys might send me into a self-hate spiral, because only losers drop their keys. Catastrophic thinking is the norm. But only for about ten days. Then I'm right as rain again. I can catch my sleeve on the door handle and just get on with the rest of my life, drop my keys and laugh about my butter fingers, and I can function perfectly normally.

I know I don't have it as badly as others. In fact, now that I know what it is and when it happens, I take an over-the-counter antihistamine to regulate the rise of histamines, which for me, possibly have an effect and can be quite helpful. (See your doctor before taking any medications, either over-the-counter or prescribed.) But I know other people with PMDD fly into a rage; some have taken their own lives and some have lost jobs, partners, family and friends over it. My brain fog, forgetfulness, sadness and overreaction are the symptoms that are toughest for me. It's only recently that people have started talking about PMDD, thanks to some incredible survivors who have started the conversation to de-stigmatise the condition and give support to people and partners. One of the little things that can turn into very big things due to PMDD is autocorrect. For instance, when you're trying to write *on my way* to someone quickly, but as you hit send, it changes to *octopus myopic*. Or when you write someone's name and it just becomes a series of letters that look like the periodic table. Cue fury and much keypad-mashing. But it can also be very funny. Once, I was trying to message Matt and Amy about my terrible PMDD *brain fog* and it autocorrected to *Brian frog*, so that's what we call it now. If the PMDD has kicked in and I start forgetting things and catastrophising little stuff, it's Brian Frog's fault. Giving it a name really helped to manage it and take its power away. Thanks, autocorrect! And thanks, Brian.

In writing this book, I asked Amy if she knew any funny stories about me and PMDD that I could include. Her reply sums up PMDD perfectly:

'What stage of your cycle are you up to, so I know which ones I can tell you?' she asked.

I looked at my period tracker. 'Ten days to go. I think we'll just leave it.'

My advice, for what it's worth: you are important and your mental wellbeing is imperative. If your illness is hurting your feelings and making you feel low, please see a psychologist, pain psychologist, counsellor, psychotherapist, or any qualified practitioner who can help you to manage your mental health. Just because you have a physical illness does not mean you should neglect your head and your heart. Pain can be traumatic, illness is stressful and relationships are hard when you aren't well. So take care of your head as well as your body. I need you around and I want you feeling as good as you can manage to.

6
Coping with Endo

*channelling the pain through
creative pursuits*

I'm a creative person: performing arts has always been my escape. Making stuff is my happy place and where I feel most alive. I love performing, writing and doing stand-up comedy. I make shows with my husband, Matt. Our most recent show was a comedy cabaret, *Endo Days* (formerly *Endo the Road*), which I mentioned earlier. Matt and I write songs together. He writes the music and does the arrangements, while I MC and, in *Endo Days*, I do the clowning, storytelling, making jokes and educating people about how to live well with endo – but also talking about how to forgive yourself when it all feels like it's too much. It brings people together to tell their stories and laugh in the face of their pain, but also find some solace in the knowledge that we're all in it together. It's about having fun, learning things, being very silly and having a big, cathartic singalong! It's educational, it's entertaining. It's endo-tainment!

It is physically arduous: sometimes, pre-show, I'm lying under a table in agony, wondering why the hell I put myself through the pain. But then I remember how much I love performing and making people laugh and how much it distracts me from the complete fuckery in my body. Also, I love to show the endo community they are not alone. There is always someone listening and caring. Also, we all get to wear pyjamas the whole time, so it's pretty great.

The show opens with me doing a comical burlesque routine that has me stripping down from pyjamas to lingerie and back into another pair of pyjamas. (It's called 'Stripper in Her Slippers'.) I don't want to spoil it for anyone who wants to see the show when I bring it to their town, but there may be tampon nipple tassels as part of the routine. As a plus-sized woman in her forties, I am more than happy to get a little scantily clad for a good cause. It's funny: I wouldn't have done that in my fit, hot twenties, but I reckon it's just because I give fewer fucks these days about what anyone thinks of my body. I care more about how I feel in my own skin than how I look; and I feel pretty good – happy to be alive. Or maybe it's because, after so many internal examinations, surgeries, ultrasounds, internal scans and assessments on my body, it feels like everyone has been up inside this old girl. So I don't care so much about showing a little skin. Either way, it's good for laughs.

Endo Days has a soundtrack of original songs and a couple of cheeky covers. It even has the boys in my backing band, The Jarmy Army, doing Beyonce choreography. It includes a very sweary song about being excluded from the 'Mum Club'. And one of my favourites is a dedication to all the doctors who misdiagnosed me and dismissed my pain condition as anxiety and stress; and we also have a song about the importance of believing patients when they say they're in pain. I adore performing and it gives me life. Performing about endo almost makes the pain worthwhile. Almost.

On my travels, I have met a stack of other endo friendos who create things to channel their energies into something beautiful to take the edge off the pain and ailments.

What do you do as your outlet? Do you have something to use as catharsis? Whether it's writing, making, playing, running, axe-throwing, driving, fishing, meditating, watching movies, reading, collecting stamps or playing poker – or anything else you can hyper-fixate on – it's good to have something that stirs you. Something that makes you remember what you're passionate about. Something that can take you somewhere away from your pain – even for a moment – and give you a break. And let you live again.

Making art: Maddy and Jamila

Artist and entrepreneur Maddy Connors is a proud Yorta Yorta, Dja Dja Wurrung and Gamilaroi woman living with endo. (You met her back in Chapter Four.) Prolific on social media, passionate about culture and causes, and an absolute joy to chat with, Maddy used the Covid-19 lockdown to pour her energies into her art and launch her business Yarli Creative, which has gone gangbusters ever since.

'I have been an artist my entire life. I was very creative as a child. I would create not only physical art, in terms of drawings and paintings, but I also would write stories,' she says. 'I started creating Yarli in the first lockdown. And because I was also on maternity leave, I had that space to create. I wanted to build my brand and my business so that I could just go back two to three days a week in the corporate world, because this is my passion. Aboriginal health is also my passion, so I wanted to keep those two together.'

Maddy says her art has been an outlet for her. It helps with her endo pain and associated symptoms, even acting as an inspiration for some of her artwork.

'I have suffered with really bad anxiety and depression my entire life. I have been a victim of family violence from a young age, and so that trauma still lies deep within me. I think art has been a way to release some of those traumas and some of the experiences that I've had. I also think that it's been able to ground me and keep me connected to my ancestors, to my culture, and to who I am spiritually,' she says. 'That connection is really amazing because it's very much like mindfulness, where you let go and you just begin to create something that you want to release from your mind to the paper or to the digital medium.'

Maddy's art is breathtakingly beautiful and tells important stories. I bought a piece from her; a painting of a uterus called Winyar, which means 'woman' in Yorta Yorta. It represents women as life-givers, nourishers and protectors, our bodies strong, resilient and enduring unparalleled pain which makes our power unsurpassed.

'With the Winyar piece, I used that as a way to send my body positivity. I used feminine and earthy colours to tie in with connecting to the earth, connecting to oneself, and trying to remove that pain. I did, however, include the blood in the image. I still wanted to reflect that pain that we feel as endo warriors, but then I also wanted it to be something that brings joy, as well.'

After talking to Maddy, I wanted to find out what other people with chronic pain do as a creative outlet, which can help manage pain and low mood. We heard from Jamila Main earlier about their experiences as a non-binary person living with endometriosis. Jamila is an actor, writer and theatre-maker. Like Maddy, they find the arts a positive outlet for their condition.

'The only time in my life I'm not in pain is when I'm performing,' Jamila says. 'When I'm in a creative development, I experience reduced pain while writing and discussing the play. I think for performance, my mind is so focused on what I have to do, my body deprioritises the pain.'

Keep finding your joy

Michelle Neilsen is a nutritionist and PPEP Talk® endo educator who has a passion for healthy living and wellbeing. She finds her creative joy in cooking and movement, which help her to manage her condition.

'I love to cook, and when I get in the zone and am whipping up tasty treats and dancing around the kitchen, it takes my mind off my pain,' she says. 'I'm able to get creative and cook delicious anti-inflammatory meals that I know are going to reduce my pain in the long run, and also incorporate fun dance movements into cooking – while also singing poorly and loudly – which helps to relax my pelvic muscles. Good food, dancing and music energises me when I'm feeling fatigued and low.'

I have been privy to Michelle's food and it is pretty spectacular. The idea of it inspiring dance is adorable and awesome. These are great outlets.

Adriana is an actor, but she has moved into directing because it's easier on her body. She finds that, while performing and directing doesn't ease her pain at all, it's a distraction because it's something she loves.

'The pain makes the anxiety higher when I need to perform or rehearse. Directing is easier, which is why I'm moving into that space. At the end of the day, you can take painkillers and sit with a heat pack and still direct. Performing is hard, especially if you have to do work in your undies and be sexy. But, of course, often when you're actually onstage and in character you can sort of forget about the pain and fall in a heap later,' she says.

For performer, teacher and director Claire, pain is difficult to ignore – but her commitment to her craft is such that she pushes through.

'Generally, I'd say ninety per cent of the time, performing makes the pain much worse. However, because of my passion and desire to perform, direct and make theatre, I'll commit more time to preparing for when I have to do it,' she says. 'I will stay in bed all day in order to be able to perform or attend my shows at night. If I have to be at rehearsals all day, full-time, I need to take painkillers, have my hot water bottle available, lie down during break times and have someone drop me off and pick me up. I guess my love of it makes my determination greater. But when I've rehearsed all week, I won't be able to get out of bed for the whole weekend afterwards.'

We need to keep up the things we love doing, even if it's a modified version. I used to be a full-time teacher, which I loved, but I had to give it up due to the physical demands it made on me. Secondary schools have a lot of stairs. Teachers are often carrying books, papers, equipment and resources to seven different classrooms in one day, standing up to teach and moving around on yard duties or sport supervision.

One school I worked at removed all of the teacher desks in every classroom because they wanted their staff to be 'on' at all times: to be active, available to students and moving around the classroom. This was absolutely exhausting, not to mention ableist, unreasonable and demoralising. It also meant students couldn't come up to the front of the classroom and have a private conversation with the teacher or seek help quietly. One wonders whether management only cared about teachers looking lively for principal tours.

These days, rather than work in schools, I run workshops with young people and adults to satisfy my love of teaching. And sometimes I take short-term contracts in schools when they become available. I learned post-diagnosis that when I stopped doing what I loved, I felt lost and sad. I don't want that for myself or my family, so I do what I can when I can, and keep living my life to the fullest. (Or the medium-est – whichever is easiest!)

I don't want to be married to this illness and I refuse to let it dictate what I do. It's a condition, not a lifestyle. So, I keep writing. I perform stand-up because it's only five to ten minutes of actual standing up – and I often use a walking stick to lean on. I clown about in cabaret shows about endo. I present a breakfast radio show every week. And I spend time with my gorgeous little family, who make me laugh and distract me from my pain. And sometimes we laugh at my illness . . . because there's nothing funnier than chronic pain, amirite? (No.)

But the humour you find in difficult situations can be the best kind. Like when you start giggling in science class during a test, or cracking up at a wedding (or funeral), or using dark humour to defuse a difficult situation with people you love.

Endo stories: sharing and processing through art

As well as continuing to do what you love, it's crucial to keep talking about endo, periods, menstrual health and everything else associated with them. We need to normalise them so we can find safety and wellness in our everyday lives. Using her visual art as a talking point, along with her stories, Maddy wants people to feel comfortable and safe to talk about their bodies and share their experiences.

'The thing that I've been getting from people is that they're feeling a strong connection, not only to my images, but also to the stories. I'm a storyteller, so my images and my creativity doesn't just come out in the form of the art. It comes out as a form of both the story and the art together. They are one, and they're in my mind and I need to people to see those, but I also do want people to have their own interpretation,' she says.

'I want people to realise that female health is not a taboo subject. It's not a subject we should hide. It's something we should talk about more with our friends and our family, and even with our partners; I think it needs to be a more open dialogue.'

Solomon Kammer is an artist who creates beautiful, confronting, award-winning paintings. Solomon is a neurodivergent health advocate and visual storyteller living with endometriosis on Kaurna Land. I knew them by reputation and when I finally had the chance to meet them, we got along famously. Disarming, sincere, whip-smart and tough as nails, Solomon has been a finalist in prestigious art competitions such as the Ramsay Prize, Shirley Hannan National Portrait Award, Kennedy Art Prize and Wyndham Art Prize and the coveted Archibald Prize, for which Jamila Main was the subject of the piece.

When Solomon first received their diagnosis of endo, they were completely broken by it and couldn't reconcile themself with it. This was the catharsis for creating the work that propelled them into the spotlight as an advocate and someone with something very important to say about chronic pain, illness and the lack of awareness surrounding it.

'When I first got my diagnosis, I dropped off the planet for three months and stayed home. I was depressed and couldn't deal with the fact that I had an incurable condition I would have forever. I didn't have any information on it at all from the doctor, and information online and the communities weren't as strong as they are now. I just didn't know what it all meant,' Solomon says.

'I got up one day after being almost catatonic and I thought, *fuck this, I've got to express myself.* I was so emotional and I couldn't put it anywhere, so I made this enormous painting of a woman with blood all over her and it was really cathartic. It took a month to paint her and it slowed everything down. All I thought about was getting my feelings out.'

The painting, *Endometriosis (Coagulate)*, turned out to be a significant painting in Solomon's career. It was published all over the media, starting big conversations about the condition.

'I wasn't trying to make a big statement but apparently I did,' Solomon says. 'I had an influx of people making contact with me and I realised I was not the only one feeling isolated and living with this thing no one understands. From that I was inspired to dive deeper into the issue, to keep talking about it and being public about the social issues around endo, as well as the fact that it was also hard for me. But also why no one was talking about it and why no one understands it, not even doctors and specialists. I was angry and motivated to uncover the issues.'

Channelling illness into artwork, Solomon initially sought comfort, but now finds empowerment, an outlet and advocacy for social change through the work they create.

'In the beginning when I was in so much pain, my art was therapeutic, but now it's become more of a political investigation. It doesn't provide me much healing anymore, but it did its job in the first place to heal me enough to get to the next stage where I feel empowered,' Solomon says.

'Or sometimes I feel angry and channel that into empowerment and action. So now it doesn't have the effect of calming me down, it has the opposite. The more I make work about it, the angrier I get about how slow the progress is with endo and with medicalisation, and how people are treated, in general. With each painting I do, it doesn't feel like enough, because I know too much now. I'm always thinking about the next painting and what I can investigate and bring to the surface.'

Endo Days: how I turned my illness into art and laughs

Matt and I started writing shows after our first pregnancy loss, because we didn't really know what else to do. We were going out a lot, but then I had caesarean surgery to remove part of a very decayed and infected uterus. So all of a sudden, we had to stay home.

We watched a lot of television. Like, a lot. Then one night, when I was well enough to enjoy wine again, Matt brought out the guitar and we started improvising parody songs about the telly shows we were watching at the time. (*Game of Thrones, Mad Men, Breaking Bad, Homeland* and other shows circa 2013.) We were making ourselves laugh so hard and one of us (we can't remember which one) suggested we turn the songs into a cabaret show. The rest is history. I overcame severe and debilitating stage fright, as well as some Grade A imposter syndrome, to put that show on a tiny little stage at a pub. But it was the start of me writing comedy to heal my heart, body and mind. After *Box Set Blues* came shows like *Something Borrowed, Something Blues; The Vinyl Club; Endo The Road; Endo Days; Extra Curricular* – and even a kids show, *For Kids About To Rock.*

When I am performing, writing, creating, or doing something else I love, I am more likely to find energy to push through the pain and discomfort. When my brain isn't focusing on muscle spasms, cramps and my various aches and pains, I can accomplish many things.

People often tell me I should slow down and stop taking on so much. I admit I take on far more than I should, and sometimes it causes great amounts of stress. But I like to grab life with two hands and take every opportunity that comes my way (also explained by my ADHD which makes me need to work on twenty projects at a time). I do this partly because I spent my years before my endo diagnosis thinking my life would be short due to my unexplained conditions. (I felt like I was dying most of the time so it definitely had to be some kind of exotic illness I picked up in the jungles of Papua New Guinea, which would surely and tragically take me by the time I was thirty – it's not. It's endo. But I did get malaria when I lived in Papua New Guinea, so it wasn't entirely implausible and over-dramatic.)

But for the most part, I do this because I know when I fill my life with things that matter to me, my body is less tense, because my muscles are more relaxed, my mind is focused on things that bring me joy and I am channelling those feelings into my passions. Of course, the condition is still there. But for those glorious moments, it is slightly numbed and pushed to the back of my life, enabling me to do things that make me feel invincible.

This is much easier said than done. If your passion is horse riding or doing squats at the gym, you will probably need to double the pelvic stretches and visits to the physio. And if what you love doing starts to cause you too much pain, you might be able to find another way of being around your 'thing' and soaking in its culture while keeping yourself safe: like coaching, documenting, commentating, teaching or promoting.

Maddy referred to her art as mindfulness. And mindfulness and meditation can help release tension and lessening muscle pain caused by endo. So, find your joy – whether it's knitting, gardening, painting pet rocks, or collecting toenail clippings. It can't hurt to channel your passions and keep your mind and body healthy.

7

Endo Friendos, Support Groups and Community

Along my chronic pain journey, I have made many friends that I fondly refer to as 'endo friendos'. Before my diagnosis, I was very social and loved being around people. But I found it difficult to commit to close friendships or relationships. I was always afraid I would let people down, or that the vague mental health condition I was diagnosed with might drive them away.

Now I know what's wrong with me, I've been able to find many more things that are right with me, too. I've been a better friend to myself and others, and I've let go of those people who gave me a hard time about being unable to attend events, or were unwilling to be patient about my occasional lack of energy and ability. That's liberating.

I highly recommend making room in your life for advocates and allies by releasing the critics and cynics. It's painful enough to live with this illness. You don't need people's negativity and judgement on top of it.

Throughout my life pre-diagnosis, I met only a few people with endometriosis. A couple of them told me they thought I had it too (though doctors disagreed). So it took me a while to find a community.

Donna Ciccia, co-founder and board director of Endometriosis Australia, says she didn't find out one of her closest friends had endo until their thirty-year school reunion. That shows how isolating it can be if we don't talk about it.

'I was talking to one of my friends who was in my class, and she said, 'You do realise the reason I never was at school was because I had endometriosis?' We were in the same class, we had two full days together every week and I still didn't even know that she had endometriosis. It wasn't something that we talked about or discussed; it just wasn't a thing. I think you bury it; you push it down; you just suck it up and just keep going,' she says.

Endo friendos: my best endo friend

Australian statistics cite the incidence of endometriosis in people who menstruate as one in nine. And birds of a feather seem to flock together. When I worked in Tammy Franks' state parliament office, three out of four of us had the condition. And at the co-working and creative education hub I run in Adelaide, Vault 134, it's four out of six. Once we find each other and the cat is out of the bag, there is no holding back on period talk, pain complains and quality uterus jokes.

One of those hilarious co-workers is Amy, who is my best mate, my work colleague, and someone who has promised to clear my browser history if I die suddenly. She and I created our co-working space together and have built an environment that is inclusive, safe and supportive, particularly to all the people with pain and endo.

Amy was diagnosed when she was about twenty and was told to have children by the time she was twenty-five, or she'd never be able to have any. She followed instructions and has three children: Evan, Mal and a four-year-old boy in her care. (Gentle reminder that not all endo patients have fertility issues and this doctor was very wrong to panic her into having children. That said, they are pretty great children.)

I can't remember how Amy and I found out we both have endo. We've been friends for a decade, have shared an office for years as freelancers and collaborated on many projects together. We've learned to schedule work around our menstrual cycles. But when we can't do that, we do everything we can to prop the other up to get through the high pain days and the low mood weeks.

'You would think sharing an office with someone who also has endo might be a bit miserable, especially as we can never seem to get our cycles to sync so, more often than not, one of us is experiencing some kind of negative symptom on most days,' Amy says. 'However, it's incredibly freeing sharing a workspace with someone who you don't have to explain why you are dressed in your stretchiest clothes ten days a month to make room for your extended belly, and for the camaraderie when you have to put on a fake smile for a half-hour meeting and then feel like you need a ten-hour nap afterward.

'And it's helpful to share stashes of drugs when you have swapped handbags and accidentally left your Ponstan or ibuprofen at home. It's great having someone who understands that some days your uterus feels so big, you can't bend over to pick something up so you just kick it under your desk for a better uterus day.'

It's true. She kicks a lot of shit under her desk. I don't reckon she's going to pick it up, either. Actually, I don't think either of us will.

'I think the best part of sharing an office with an endo friendo is that we accept and respect the tired, stressed and emotional Endo Amy and Endo Libby as much as the well and pain-free sides of each other,' she says.

'Sometimes those two sides of us seem like two different people to non-sufferers, but we understand that while the stressed and sensitive endo flare-up sides of us aren't always pleasant or as rational as we might always like, we never say things like, *you are over-reacting because you are in pain/hormonal/tired.* We accept and treat each other's high and lows and respect each other's rights to have a meltdown over an imagined slight, or a cry over hurt feelings that may not be as big a deal when we are feeling good. That radical acceptance is really hard to find.'

I would be lost without Amy's support and enabling behaviour (she is the master of twisting my arm to leave work early to go to the pub or go get our nails done). She gives me the space to be a hormonal banshee and will heat up a wheat bag if I'm cramping, so I can get through a gig or a day of meetings. And we never compare pain or dismiss each other's symptoms.

'Don't get me wrong, I'm still going to gently ask how many days until your period is due, or recommend some endo self-care, but it's never used as a way to dismiss your reactions and feelings,' she says.

Because of the shame attached to my illness after years of humiliation and misdiagnosis, I have found safety and comfort in associating with 'my own kind'. Amy can sometimes see my symptoms before I do and she will tell me to slow down, or she'll find a way to make things easier for me, and vice versa. We work for ourselves, partly due to illness and partly due to a mutual dislike for being told what to do. We do have clients to report to, though, so having each other's support has been beneficial to our businesses as well as our physical and mental health. She's also excellent to share a bottle of wine with. (But that's another story and not quite as good for our health.)

'When you have endo there are so many ways you can be gaslighted, you often end up gaslighting yourself. It's important to have a friend and a comrade who would never say you're overreacting,' Amy says. 'With friends who don't have endo, I get worried they think it's an excuse or they think I should just push through it. It's not just the pain though; it's the exhaustion and the stress of trying to tackle life, parenting and work while managing the pain.'

As Susan mentioned a few chapters ago, endo is more than just lesions. Symptoms like low mood, fatigue, nausea, fainting, vomiting, food sensitivities, and immune vulnerability can be debilitating. Amy and I use our shared knowledge and experiences of endo to get each other through the trickier times.

'It's so nice that you instantly understand all the implications of the pain, not just the pain itself,' she says. 'Like understanding the emotional labour of building yourself up to show up to things through the pain and the exhaustion and still being on top of your game for clients.'

Learning, empathising and building a community together

When Peta-Anne moved into our office, she spoke of her health concerns: painful periods, lower back pain, muscle spasms and pelvic pain. It sounded suspiciously like endo to us, so we gently nudged her toward a gynaecologist. It turned out we were right. She has now, in her late forties, had an excision, hysterectomy and started a treatment plan.

Of course, I don't go around diagnosing people, because endo symptoms are wildly different for everyone and they echo a few other illnesses. Not to mention the fact that I am definitely not a doctor (though I would like to wear a stethoscope and carry a clipboard to look important). But it's important to me to share the things I have learned in my endo education quest, to arm others with information and to talk about our illness.

Amy and I talk about it candidly and often, because when we talk about our pain and we talk about our condition, people might hear themselves in those words and it might lead them to have their own health checked. Even if they don't have endo, it's always worth ruling things out, because it gets you on track towards discovering the real issue. For Peta-Anne, joining the conversation with us has given her support for herself and motivation to help others.

'I've been alerted to my own endo, and there has been a camaraderie and positivity in the workplace that makes us feel we are not alone and that we're heard and seen,' she says.

My friend Jacquie introduced me to Claire because she knew we both had endo and, at the time, Claire was struggling post-surgery. You met Claire in chapter one, and she pops up quite a bit in this book.

At the time we were introduced, Claire was recovering from an excision and wasn't feeling good. She had questions and didn't know where to turn. Going to specialists is expensive and it can take a while to get an appointment. Sometimes online groups can get a bit noisy when you're feeling sensitive. Claire was seeking some comfort, conversation and understanding. We chatted online for ages before we actually met in person and she has become one of my very favourite people.

'Every sufferer of endo needs an endo friendo,' Claire says. 'You are my most cherished one. You have either been through what I am going through in any given moment, or you can empathise and appreciate my experiences because you live with endo yourself.

'You are the first person I talk to when I'm really struggling with pain, bleeding, mental health, grief, medical indifference, medication or any of the myriad of things I face week to week. You are there to hold my hand (virtually or in real life), to give me advice, to play me songs, feed me wine and cheese, or just to listen. Your friendship has helped me navigate this lifelong, crippling disease and I can't imagine my life without you.'

Excuse me while I have a little cry about this lovely revelation from Claire.

After keeping people at arm's length for so long because I was so frightened of being a crap friend (and also because I felt ashamed of my failing body), I have found love, comfort, peace, understanding, confidence and strength in my endo community. I've found my people, which has given me the conviction to make (and keep) friends outside the endo sphere.

Queer and trans community support

Lewis, who we chatted with earlier, says it can be difficult for trans people who are living with any sort of dysphoria or dysmorphia to find community because they might not want to discuss their bodies. But Lewis had a friend who was able to find a way to discuss it without causing distress.

'I had a conversation with my friend where I just said, *I've got pain.*

It's something pressing against my stomach. And they said, *I know what that is, but I'm not going to say unless you want me to.* It was actually quite polite of them not to just go, *This is the diagnosis,'* Lewis says.

'A while later I asked what they thought it was and they said, *it's probably endometriosis,* so I got a referral and the process of diagnosis began.'

Lewis says their friendships in the queer community have led to finding trans-friendly, safe spaces to seek medical assistance, which is the best way to land yourself with a medical cheer squad you can trust and rely upon.

Online support groups

Kara* (fifteen) lives in rural South Australia (Narungga) and says she relies on the online community because it's too hard to find a safe and engaged community in her home town. Kara preferred not to use her real name.

'I am part of a lot of online worlds because my family don't know I'm queer and they don't really like hearing about my endo because periods are disgusting to them,' she says. 'But I can escape through forums and groups where it's okay to be who I am, to talk about my endo and get advice from people because I'm not getting any at home. I've made some good friends through it and I'm going to meet them when I move to Adelaide after I've finished school.'

When I received my endo diagnosis in 2014, I joined all the online support groups. Every single one. And then, one by one, I left them all. I wasn't ready for the onslaught of posts. It was a bit overwhelming and quite scary. One afternoon when I was having a high pain day and was feeling vulnerable, the group administrator of a Facebook support group for endo posted something like, 'This is a support group and none of you are giving me any support. If you don't reply to this post by midnight tonight, I am banning you all!'

As I slowly backed away from the computer, I thought, *are all groups as wild as this?* Spoiler: they're not.

As I started to accept my fate a bit more, I re-joined some of them (not the one with the dictator admin) and read thread after thread of conversations, queries and complaints. It was entertaining, excruciating, informative, educational, and actually a very good use of my time. I stayed in the groups that are moderated well, and take the time and effort to look after their members.

There are different endo support groups that will suit different people, depending on your needs for a safe and supportive space. I can't be in groups that have a lot of drama and online arguing, so I steer clear of most of the heavily populated global groups and stick with ones that are more relevant to my own location and needs. While it's interesting to see what's going on overseas, some of the global groups have so many members, which is difficult to moderate, leading to fights, inappropriate advice, repetitive posts, MLM (multi-level marketing/pyramid schemes) sales and drug shaming (where someone disapproves of your treatment and harasses you for it). Online aggro gives me heart palpitations. Reading comment sections on Facebook can often be an exercise in self-harm.

I was once blocked on Facebook by someone who I met through a support group. She was having trouble getting pregnant. She contacted me many times a day and it was clear she was in a deep depression about it. I talked with her, listened, shared stories, offered (not medical) advice and, in the end, she blocked me because I had a second ectopic pregnancy and she said, 'At least you can get pregnant.'

I hope she is going okay and I am sorry she felt hurt, but in the end, it was very much a one-way friendship that ended in a giant slap in the face when I was at a pretty low point. From that experience, I am learning to try to ensure that people have the mental capacity to take on my issues before I share them and I will do the same with them. I don't always get it right, but I try to be more aware now.

I have quite a few mates I have met through online support groups and it's a fabulous way to socialise without leaving the house. It's also instant support when you need it. But remember to make sure you give as much support and attention as you receive.

Donna Ciccio: Endometriosis Australia

Through my work in the Australian Coalition for Endometriosis, I had the good fortune of getting to know some of the people involved in endometriosis support groups. Each one shared a similar story of being diagnosed, looking for help, having to help themselves and then wanting to pass on that knowledge to others. Most of them are volunteers, who are very dedicated to endo awareness and education.

Donna Ciccia was diagnosed in 2001. Like me (with Dr Susan Evans), she was fortunate to find an expert who helped her navigate the process, Professor Jason Abbott (the surgeon and farmer we spoke with earlier). Unlike me, though, she didn't have an online network to lean on – so she started Endometriosis Australia with Jason, who has now been her doctor and colleague for two decades.

'When I was younger, I was in emergency with every period. I couldn't function and I was just very blessed that I had a friend whose sister-in-law was a nurse at Randwick Women's, and that's how I was diagnosed. Jason was my doctor. I was very, very lucky,' she says.

In the early 2000s, the pair were lamenting the lack of resources and support during one of their consultations. It was Donna's idea to start a national organisation.

'It took us about four years to get it up and running,' says Jason. 'It has been very much a labour of love and it's all about the patient voice and working towards an end to the suffering.'

The key principles of Endometriosis Australia have always been around education and awareness, as well as raising funds for research. Its passion project is now funding programs for patients, researchers and specialists across Australia. Endometriosis Australia has been instrumental in putting endometriosis on parliamentary agendas, at both state and federal levels.

Donna says she put her own health second to build Endometriosis Australia. She estimates she spent around eighty to one hundred hours a week working on the association.

'That's what it's like in small NFPs [not-for-profit organisations]: you are it. You've got to be the jack of all trades and do everything. Now, I'm trying to stop on weekends and have that as my time, but it's hard,' she says.

And while Jason is busy being a gynaecologist, laparoscopic surgeon, professor and farmer (I can't quite move on from that, as you can see!), he has devoted a huge amount of energy to working with Donna to create a safe space for people living with endo. Jason says the driving goal of Endometriosis Australia is to offer endo sufferers somewhere to talk about it, and to promote awareness of all aspects of endometriosis.

'I continue to be in awe of what has been achieved by, effectively an organisation with no real income, that has developed a small stream of charitable events and sourcing money from the very people who are suffering with the disease,' he says.

Jess Taylor: QENDO

Jess Taylor is president of QENDO, Queensland's online and in person support group for endo. The moment she was diagnosed, she threw herself into helping people. She wasn't given any guidance or information and she became frustrated and angry, wondering what support was available for people like her.

'I was so scared,' she remembers of her diagnostic laparoscopy. 'No one spoke with me through that whole process or told me what to expect. I was going in for this operation that no one explained to me, and when I looked anything up, the words weren't making any sense.'

She was about to create her own group, after a few false starts and many dead ends, before she found one in her area. As she was working through the process of developing a charity, she came across QENDO, which had then been around for twenty years.

'I spoke with the then president, for a very long time,' she recalls. 'It was the first and only time anyone ever actually listened to me, and heard me as a person.'

Jess was relieved and more than a little excited to get on board.

'Learning about their support and services, I said, *Sign me up! Sign me up! I am doing this, I am a part of this!*' she laughs. 'I said, *We need to inject some fun into this, we're going to have a ladies' night fundraiser, with a fashion parade, expensive cars, and we're going to have some fun; we're going to do it in six weeks' time.* I just told this committee what we were going to do, and they freaked out.'

Jess made that event happen. They filled the whole street, emptied the ATMs and showed people affected by endo that there is help and support available to them.

Her dedication to helping people with endo has been tireless. She led a team to develop the QENDO app, which is a hub of support in your pocket. They also developed a phone service you can call if you are ever feeling lost, scared or alone in anything endo related (1800 ASK QENDO), and a range of other resources. They are all available to all endo patients and supporters all across Australia. Jess leads a team of passionate people who are making a difference to those with the condition.

'People who are diagnosed have so many questions, like how do I talk about this to my partner? How do I talk about this to my mum? How do I communicate this with my team of medical people who I now need to find? Who do I talk to? What is genuine information? What isn't?'

The QENDO app is a support hub that invites users to log their journey and offers tips on how to communicate various things with doctors and specialists, or natural therapists – whatever path you choose according to your needs. It teaches people to understand their condition.

'From diagnosis on, they have actual credible information and they're not left searching for five, ten hours through these Facebook groups that aren't monitored, that are only anecdotal experiences,' says Jess. 'Those experiences are really valid, but patients need more than that to navigate the early days of an endo diagnosis.'

Yeah, that was me. Hours and hours of trying to sift through anecdotes to find fact-based or Australian-based research. An app or a website would have been great. Or just something that said, *Hi, welcome to your disease. This is the rest of your life! Please enjoy the buffet breakfast*. And then offered me a whole lot of really helpful information, options and croissants.

A new kid on the block is EndoZone, which is a website acting as a one-stop shop for all your endo needs. It's for patients, supporters and medical professionals and can be found at endozone.com.au. EndoZone was built in consultation with endo patients, the medical community and all of the national support groups. I helped work on the platform and was part of the consultation process where they reached out to the endo community with surveys, focus groups and beta testing, to make sure it was built for endo people *by* endo people. QENDO did the same kind of consultation with their app. (I muscled my way into that one as well.)

Each group has their own culture, values, and mission. And while you can choose one and stick with it, every group is doing something different and innovative, so it's good to check out what they all have on offer. There are plenty of endo influencers on social media too, who share really interesting tips and tricks for living with the illness. To find them, follow hashtags like #endo #endometriosis #endolife and #endowarrior on your favourite social media sites. It doesn't matter where you get your information from, so long as you are able to find evidence-based advice and a safe space for you.

Syl and Lesley Freedman: EndoActive

Mother-and-daughter team Syl and Lesley Freedman started EndoActive to collate and create a user-friendly, centralised system for endometriosis information and research. I've had the privilege of working with this dynamic duo on ACE projects.

Syl, now twenty-nine, was given her endo diagnosis at twenty-one years old. Then – surprise surprise – she felt lost and confused about where to go next. (Are you sensing a theme here?)

'My frustration was increasing that I was having all these different problems and I couldn't get help at just one place, one clinic under one roof,' Syl says. 'I honestly felt like I was going to a different specialist five days a week, and I just didn't have the energy for it. It was so expensive and so annoying. I just felt like my life was just a revolving door of doctor's waiting rooms with not much very good advice.'

Then Syl's mum, Lesley, got her hands on the abstracts of the Australasian Gynaecological Endoscopy and Surgery (AGES) society congress and they found out about Visanne, a drug that was being used overseas (but not in Australia) to treat endometriosis. Visanne contains a progestogen hormone, dienogest, which shrinks endometrial tissue and can help reduce pelvic pain and painful periods. The beginning of EndoActive was their Change. Org petition to demand pharmaceutical giant Bayer bring the drug into Australia. It was approved for use here, but Bayer didn't think there was enough demand and that it wouldn't be financially viable. (Refresher: one in nine people who menstruate have endometriosis. No demand? Hmm, righto.)

Lesley contacted Bayer to get the ball rolling and had some friends sign the petition. Then Syl decided to take it online.

'I didn't have a clue how to manage an online platform,' Lesley recalls. 'We learned quite quickly. It became a challenge for me to make Bayer say yes, because I just I can't be bothered with companies who will put a drug in some countries and not others.

Particularly since it had already been to the TGA (Therapeutic Goods Administration), so I knew it had approval.'

Within six weeks, they had 74,500 signatures and 19,000 comments. Bayer agreed to release Visanne in Australia. Then the pair started reading the comments on the petition and realised there were others like them who were alone and seeking help, so they started EndoActive, a platform for support and activism.

'I wondered what we could do with the momentum we had gathered,' Lesley says. 'And because my business is to make training videos, and there were so many people looking for information, what we needed was an explainer video or DVD.'

Through EndoActive, they make educational videos and resources about endo, which are free to the community, covering topics such as pelvic physio, mindfulness, pelvic pain, central sensitisation, bowel health and so much more valuable information, which is available on their website. But before they developed this wealth of knowledge, they were grasping, just like so many of us.

EndoActive has been a labour of love for Syl and Lesley. It has given as much to them as it has given to the endo community.

'There have been times when Syl and I have felt very low, but there was always so much to do and so many other people worse off. And so many people that we felt we could help,' Lesley says.

Syl says, 'For me, EndoActive made a huge difference to my life. In the beginning it was driven by Les, because I was really sick. Managing the Facebook page was the job I gave myself. It was my way of starting to get back into some type of work, because I hadn't been able to work in a really long time. I was just too unreliable and sick all the time.

'It meant I had something to do, to be able to read people's stories, even if I was in bed, sick. It gave me a sense of purpose again, because I felt so useless. And then were getting requests from media, all the time. So, it really became more than a full-time job. There was a couple of years, or a few years, where we would work on EndoActive seven days a week. You couldn't just leave the Facebook page for a day because there was just so much activity. I would keep managing and monitoring it even when I was out with friends.'

Managing an online community is a lot of work: I know this. Endometriosis patients are a huge population across Australia and the world. People are newly diagnosed every day.

'I still adore EndoActive,' Syl says. 'I don't want to give it up, because it has been such a big part of my identity. I feel way prouder at a dinner party if people are like, *What do you do?* And I say, *I'm a part of this amazing thing that helps people, it's high job satisfaction and it means a lot*, rather than saying I just do some regular job.'

Vanessa, Meike and me: Endometriosis Support SA

In 2014, the first group I found online was Endometriosis Australia. But I was looking for something closer to home. I didn't know anyone with endometriosis. But because it affects one in nine people who menstruate, I figured it wouldn't be long before I found some company. (Especially as Adelaide is a small place and we all seem to know someone who knows someone who knows us!)

I met Vanessa and Meike, founders of Endometriosis Support SA, at an Endometriosis Australia EndoMarch High Tea. We quickly became friends.

At thirty-two, dentist Dr Vanessa Platt was diagnosed with endometriosis after a GP told her she'd just pulled a muscle. She demanded an ultrasound, but the doctor refused until she insisted. It showed a burst ovarian cyst.

A week later, her pain became so bad she was taken for emergency laparoscopic surgery, where she was diagnosed with endo.

'I woke up from the surgery and the doctor said, *You've got stage-four endo* and I said, *What's endo?* My pain didn't get much better after that,' she says. 'In the end, it was so bad, I literally couldn't function. It was just so horrendous, and I knew that I didn't want any more children. At thirty-five, I decided to have a hysterectomy.'

Vanessa, a funny, energetic and charismatic, British-born health practitioner, says she knows a hysterectomy isn't the solution for everyone. 'But for me, a hysterectomy has actually worked, and my pain is so much better. I do get pelvic pain flare-ups, but that's muscle memory.'

Like all the others I spoke to who started support groups, Vanessa started the South Australian group to connect and take herself out of isolation.

'I wasn't quite sure what endo was and didn't know anyone else who had it. I really wanted to speak to somebody I could relate to, and just discuss and share ideas,' she says. 'I looked around South Australia and couldn't find anything. Then Susan (Evans) put me in touch with Meike and we decided to start our support group, because we just wanted to help other people. I wanted some good to come out of what had happened to me.

'I was lucky growing up,' she says. 'I had strong feminists around me and was told women can do anything. But that isn't the case with everyone. As we all know, it's easy for endo symptoms to get overlooked and to get fobbed off by doctors, especially being women.'

Meike has since moved on from the group and Vanessa has now handed over the reins to me. She has created a gentle and supportive culture for South Australian endo patients, which is a pleasure to run. Every day, there are new groups and initiatives popping up and I think it's awesome – the more the better!

Some people don't like the rules in the groups they find, so they start their own. Some people would prefer their groups with a focus on older or younger people, so they create a group to suit their stage of life.

Rather than feel threatened by other endo groups, we should embrace them all. We are all on the same team, kicking in the same direction – but our needs and personalities are different to each other and that should be reflected in our support groups. As long as you're getting factual information and genuine rallying and support, it doesn't matter what your cheer squad looks like.

'People just need the right tools,' says Vanessa. 'Holistic care isn't just about finding the right doctor. It's everything else. It's health, diet, exercise, physio and complementary medicine, as well as conventional medicine. And emotional support too, including making sure you can access support from family and friends. You need a whole care package, a whole guide, because it's not just one discipline.'

Without volunteers like Vanessa, I'd still be running around in the dark bumping into walls, feeling lonely and wondering what the hell is wrong with me. Our volunteers are the ones storming the barricades, approaching parliament to demand reform, creating educational programs and resources, selling useful products to aid with pain relief, developing apps, running phone lines and coming up with ways to continue to keep us connected. Most states and territories have their own consumer groups working overtime every day and night.

Dr Susan Evans and me: Pelvic Pain Foundation of Australia

It took me a little while to learn to accept this condition and forgive myself. But after accepting my diagnosis, Dr Susan Evans (who would co-write PPEP Talk® with me) was one of my first endo friendos. With all the knowledge and contacts she'd accumulated, as author of *Endometriosis and Pelvic Pain* and chair of Pelvic Pain Australia, Susan introduced me to a dynamic group of people who are still fighting, lobbying, educating and pushing to get endometriosis on the agenda. This group of superheroes was the Australian Coalition for Endometriosis (ACE), which comprises endo consumer bodies and associations from around Australia, researchers, patients, doctors, and politicians. I spent some time on ACE and wow, did I learn a lot! This group of spectacular people are working for endo patients to raise awareness, spread the word, support people, develop resources and keep you connected. And, a lot of the time, they're doing it voluntarily, while they're living with (or treating) endo. I'll introduce you to some of those people throughout the book. You'll love them.

I value all of the people I have met along my endo journey who have either become my confidantes and shoulders to cry on, my medical cheer squad, my colleagues in the work towards awareness, education and reform; or fellow soldiers in the fight against inequality in research and medicine. Menstrual and reproductive health has a very long way to go before we are anywhere near equal in treatment and care. I often wonder whether men would be so readily dismissed or misdiagnosed if they went to a doctor about pelvic pain. (But I think I know the answer to that.)

Those who are applying for research grants, investigating new treatments and methods, developing digital platforms and building online support centres are in a difficult business. The health of people assigned female at birth should be far better resourced and better funded.

Susan told me that, despite endo surgery being difficult, she was determined to become highly skilled in this area to change people's lives and help them to live well. She's continued to be one of the foremost specialists in the condition.

'I decided as soon as I got my bit of paper that I didn't want to be an obstetrician. Gynae was where it was at, and laparoscopic surgery was my future,' she says. 'That would have been September '96. I started in private practice and my aim was to be the best laparoscopic surgeon I could possibly be.

'I worked really hard at developing and getting as good as I could. And when you do difficult laparoscopic surgery, you end up doing a lot of endometriosis, because endo is the hardest laparoscopic surgery. And if you do endo, you see a lot of people in pain. Back in the '90s, we had this concept that if we could just get a surgery right, then we could fix pain.'

Through her learning and development as a surgeon, Susan realised it wasn't that simple, which piqued her interest in discovering more. She realised there was a lot more to pain than what she was removing at an operation. It was at this point she made the decision to pass on some of her knowledge to patients to educate, inform and empower them.

'I started to study a lot outside gynaecology, looking for different specialties and what they had to contribute to pelvic pain,' she says.

She published her book. Then she realised there was a gap in support and representation, and launched Pelvic Pain Foundation of Australia to further her work as an advocate for people living with pain.

I spent a few years as a director on the PPFA board. And with PPFA, I lobbied state and federal governments for funding for PPEP Talk®. I'd never been on a board before: the imposter syndrome was real. For most of my life, my poor health was a source of frustration, embarrassment and confusion for me. Now, I was being asked to use it to contribute to an organisation working to improve things for people like me. I used my skills in media and communications and education, as well as my connections in schools and parliament, to throw myself into the PPEP Talk® project. At a time where I was trying to have a baby and kept suffering losses, it was a welcome distraction and a positive outlet.

Endo politics

Federal Liberal MP Nicolle Flint was one of a bipartisan team I worked with, across state and federal parliament, to establish the National Action Plan for Endometriosis, which included funding for endometriosis education. (Others included Katrine Hildyard MP, Tammy Franks MLC, Minister John Gardner, Minister Stephen Wade, Minister Greg Hunt, Gai Brodtmann MP and Nola Marino MP.)

Though Nicolle and I have different politics, we formed a friendship through our common drive to get endometriosis recognised and funded.

'I'm now up to forty-four women from my personal and professional network who have endo,' she told me in 2020. 'I've always been so passionate about it, because I just get so angry that women have been completely and utterly mistreated, ignored and marginalised by the medical profession.'

Nicolle joined forces with former Labor MP Gai Brodtmann, and Liberal MP Nola Marino (whose daughter suffered terribly with endo) and launched the Parliamentary Friends of Endometriosis, which included the endo groups and individuals that now also form the Australian Coalition of Endometriosis (ACE), on which I also spent some time.

I was with ACE when we advised Minister Hunt on the National Action Plan for Endometriosis. Standing alongside fierce and passionate people advocating for change was electric: one of the best things I've ever been part of. If you are angry and passionate about change, I recommend joining a lobby group. It's a good way to channel your fury into something positive for yourself and others. Feels good.

While she was working to help us, Nicolle discovered that she, too, suffered from the very illness she was fighting for.

'That's the problem, when you're still soldiering on and you don't know that pain isn't normal,' she says. 'We've got to get people diagnosed sooner. We have so much more to do, in terms of communicating to women what the symptoms are.'

I often think about how privileged I was to work with friends who could change my life and my health so profoundly. One of the best things about my eventual diagnosis was finding my cheer squad – a group of people who just got it; who got *me*.

Finding a crew who can empathise with your pain and problems is a positive thing to do. There are plenty of online support groups, so you don't even have to leave the comfort of your couch to get your dose of sympathy. There are Facebook groups, Instagram accounts, websites, phone lines, in-person meet-ups, all to help you find your people. EndoZone is a good place to start if you want an updated list of resources. I have listed some in the back of the book but this is a growing and evolving space, so jump online and see what new groups and organisations are out there to meet your needs.

Community, cabaret and *Endo Days*

Community has also been my favourite feature of my cabaret show, *Endo Days*. This is something that developed organically and has become the best thing about the show. The idea came about over a few wines with Amy and my husband, Matt on the day registrations for Adelaide Fringe were closing. It was a rash, last-minute decision and we just threw in an application with plans to work out the details later. The response to the show has been both surprising and humbling – and connection has been at the heart of that.

Across four seasons, I have shared my chronic pain stories while audience members have been encouraged to share theirs in between the songs and comedy. This created a wonderfully supportive and positive atmosphere, and we have come to refer to the show as a singing support group. During the performances, we've laughed together, cried together and I've even had someone take the microphone to tell stories about her difficult sex life (no regrets, it was great for her to get it out and get some much-needed sympathy from the audience). The best thing to come out of it was feedback from people saying how inclusive, safe, supportive and educational the show was and how it gave them hope and the feeling they aren't alone. On a worryingly large number of occasions, I had endo patients come to the show and bring friends, family or partners that didn't want to acknowledge their pain or symptoms. By the end of the show, they had certainly changed their tune after hearing the voices of the people living with the condition. Strength in numbers is so powerful. That's the community I want to provide for everyone. I want patients and supporters to know I'm here, I'm listening and I believe you.

Endo friendos are the best friendos. They get it. They will accept if you cancel (because they'll do it, too), they know what you're going through and they are the best people to make gross period jokes about stained undies, blowouts in the night and period diarrhoea (when you know, you know).

I think I'm happy to end this chapter on that messy note.

5 tips for finding your endo crew:

1. Join an online support group. There are groups in every state, as well as a couple of national ones. I find the national ones to be helpful, but a little noisy for me. Finding one based in your own state will ensure you get relevant, local information that will help you.

   Before posting a question, always conduct a search of your topic in the group and read up on previous posts. This will give you a breadth of information, help you get to know who has similar issues as you. It will also ensure your post isn't removed or rejected because there have already been seven posts of 'What should I take with me to hospital?' that day.

2. Bookmark some websites like (but definitely not limited to) EndoZone, Endometriosis Australia, QENDO, EndoActive, PPFA, and Jean Hailes. They'll give you easy access to resources and information.

3. Attend endo events. The people in your endo support groups arrange events with guest speakers that are mostly free or low cost, with information about pain management, surgery, physio, medications and more. Those events are wonderful opportunities to meet friends and learn about your illness. Knowledge is power.

4. Go to the EndoMarch celebrations. Endometriosis Australia has a wonderful high tea you can attend. (And I hear there's a really fun cabaret show at Adelaide Fringe!)

5. Ask for help if you need it. This is how you will find your allies. People who lend a hand when you need it are diamonds. Treasure them.

8
Chucking Sickies

endo at work

Trigger warnings: *suicidal ideation, assault with a deadly weapon*

Having a job when you are living with a chronic illness sometimes feels impossible. For some people, it is. My chronic pain has always been cyclical, so there are some weeks where I'm feeling great; other times I feel so heavy, I can barely lift my body off the bed. At this stage of my life, I have pain on most days of the month and I care for a toddler. So working for myself has been ideal.

Before my endo diagnosis, I had no idea what to tell my employers to explain why I was sometimes a bit physically useless: I didn't actually know why either. All I knew is that I often felt unwell, heavy, in pain, dizzy, foggy and severely fatigued.

Disclosing health issues at work (Part 1)
When I was twenty-three, I fainted in a video store. (Note: video stores are an historical remnant from days past, where you stroll down the physical aisles of a Netflix menu, hire two new releases and three weeklies, and then pay an unreasonable amount of money in late fees when you forget to return them.) My partner at the time rushed me to the doctor. We both thought something was seriously wrong with me, as I had been fainting fairly regularly. But the doctor told me I had just experienced a panic attack (a physical

and mental reaction where you feel like you're dying, characterised by shortness of breath, sweating, increased heartrate, impending sense of doom). I was confused. I asked him why I would have had a panic attack in the video store. He said, 'Probably too much choice in movies.'

I recall times in the years after that diagnosis, when I was relaxing on the couch or hanging out with friends – doing pretty mundane or enjoyable things – and feeling faint, soggy in the brain, heavy in the body and generally very unwell. I'd wonder what could be causing the panic attack. I would try to breathe through it and psychoanalyse everything that had happened up until that point. It would usually end in me over-assessing every word and action, trying to find the root of the panic. On reflection, it was not a very healthy activity. But I was doing my best to treat my 'condition'.

As an aside: about a year on from the video store incident, I had an actual, real-life panic attack, the day after I was held up at knifepoint at a convenience store, by an English backpacker who was in South Australia picking fruit and ran out of money. I was working alone at the store on a Sunday morning and he came in with a kitchen knife, held it to my stomach and demanded money. He made off with about $80, a Mars Bar and a packet of cigarettes. I was left with PTSD. (He was caught directly after the incident because he'd taken the money he stole from the store and cash he'd pinched from other backpackers at the hostel and tried his luck at the casino, appearing on every CCTV along the way.) The panic attack the day after that incident snuck up on me, because I was already in a state of hypervigilance. But I remember it being completely different to the fainting I was suffering. It was definitely far more panicky and attacky.

But, back to the Great Diagnosis of the Video Store Panic Attack: I felt my best course of action was to tell my manager at the restaurant I was working at. That would be the sensible and transparent thing to do, right? I was twenty-three and totally confident that I would not be stigmatised, judged or disadvantaged as a result of my honesty about the mental health issue that was literally knocking me off my feet. What was the worst that could happen?

Well, they treated me like I was teetering on the edge of complete mental breakdown. You see, the problem is that while many people have what's colloquially known as RBF (Resting Bitch Face), I have RDF (Resting Distressed Face). So, every time I was concentrating (which was often, because carrying plates requires coordination), the manager would come up and hiss in my ear to go into the kitchen if I was going to pass out. Therefore, I had to make sure I plastered a smile onto my face for the entirety of my shift, lest I be banished to the kitchen.

This made people think I was even more unhinged, but at least they thought I was deranged and happy. It wasn't long before my shifts were cut and I had to take other work at a cafe. This job was more physically demanding. I went to yet another GP to talk about my pain and fatigue and was diagnosed with irritable bowel syndrome (IBS). I told my cafe boss and she recoiled and cried, 'Ew, gross! Don't poo on me!' (Note: pooing on people is not an actual feature of irritable bowel syndrome.)

Overloaded and exhausted at work

After that, I didn't bother to tell employers about my so-called panic disorders, IBS or any of my health issues if it were avoidable. Until I was thirty-two, working in a teaching job where my timetable was overloaded and my physical health had started to deteriorate quite significantly.

I was so tired every day and couldn't keep up with my workload. In the last week of my first term at the school, my brain fog was so bad I figured I must have a vitamin deficiency or something. So I went into a pharmacy, scooped up a stack of multivitamins and placebo energy treatments and dumped them all on the counter. My brain was tackling a thousand things that were moving slowly through the fog in my head and I forgot my PIN when I tried to pay with my card (this was before tap-and-go payments). I just completely drew a blank. I had to put my planned purchases back on the shelf and walk out, wondering what the hell had happened.

My body was weak and I felt sluggish and listless all the time – even though I was eating well and exercising at the gym every day. Physically, I was probably the fittest I'd been in my whole life, while feeling the worst I'd ever felt. But the fact that my brain forgot my PIN – four easy digits – scared me. I have a photographic memory for numbers. I have committed phone numbers, my tax file number, my uni student ID number and a whole lot of useless figures to memory.

I went to a GP and asked, in earnest, if it was possible that I had early-onset dementia. My memory was usually absolutely sharp as a tack, but my dear grandmother had just died and she had Alzheimer's. Could that be happening to me? I was scared. But my GP said I was just stressed. And I *was* stressed. My car had just broken down, my house had been broken into, my phone broke and a boyfriend I really liked had just broken up with me. Everything was, well, broken.

I made an appointment to see my boss at my school. I never took sick days at that point. Ever. I was still hanging onto a ridiculous work ethic, where illness was weakness and physical pain was just a panic attack. I pushed through every single goddamned day, even when I was at my very worst.

I loved the school I was at, adored my job and the students. I had a bunch of colleagues who were also wonderful friends. (One of those friends was Matt, who'd later become the husband you've been hearing about.) I was so proud I'd found a permanent teaching job – which isn't easy – so I was working long hours, putting everything I had into being the best teacher I could possibly be. When my health began to fail me, I was devastated. I was diagnosed with stress and depression (again) and told to quit my job (again) – but I didn't this time.

Instead, I went to the principal and said I'd have to take a step back from everything I was doing because of a debilitating mental illness. (I was teaching six English/Drama classes, running a mentor group, coordinating the student representative council/ SRC from years eight to twelve, and sitting on the staff consultative committee.) He was lovely about it. Disappointed he'd have to find someone to pick up my slack, but supportive and kind; he worked with me to decide what I might drop from my enormous workload. We agreed it would be the consultative committee and the mentor group. I was so angry with my brain for doing this in my first permanent job, which I'd worked so hard to get.

I quit all the things I was doing in my personal life that were filling the hole left by the boyfriend (producing a community television show, studying an advanced diploma in professional writing, tutoring, babysitting, going to the gym). Cutting back helped take the edge off the exhaustion, but all those symptoms were still there. Even when I wasn't stressed. I tried everything to relieve stress and combat the depression and anxiety I was told was now severe. (Exercise, psychology, mindfulness, meditation, writing poetry, baths, online dating.) But while the mental symptoms started to go away, the physical ones did not.

Keeping a job with deteriorating health

Over the course of the next two years, dating from the great Mystery of the PIN Code Brain Fart, I worked on myself and my health. I filled my life with fun, friends, family. I won a promotion and fell in love with my faculty coordinator, who I am now married to.

Things were great personally and professionally, but my health was total crap. I had crushing fatigue and moments where I just couldn't get up, even if I tried. My whole body felt as if it were full of concrete: really achy concrete. My immune system was so low, I picked up every bug that came my way (which, in a school, is a lot). At the end of that two years, I conceded my health had taken a massive tumble and I needed to drop even more things off my schedule and take a greater step back.

I went to the doctor. I was diagnosed with stress (again) but now I was starting to realise I was sick. Really sick. Physically sick. I was scared. I was living alone and most days, I would get home from work at 4:30pm and fall straight into bed, sometimes sleeping through until the next day. I was falling behind in my marking and planning, and I didn't love my job anymore: it was too hard to stay afloat. I was grumpy, tired and I felt about 150 years old. My doctor gave me a prescription for antidepressants, and advised a whole lot of vitamins and supplements.

This time, I filled the prescription for antidepressants; I was struggling and wanted any help I could get. The drugs took the edge off my low mood. But they didn't help with the physical symptoms. By now, I was starting to wake up to the fact that stress and anxiety were a lazy diagnosis and there was something else happening. I couldn't possibly feel like an enormous, mouldy sack of potatoes just because my job was a bit hectic. There were other factors at play: physical factors.

Back I went to my doctor for the fifth time in two months. I told him I'd tried all his solutions for a sick head and maybe it was time to look at my body, which seemed to be wanting to kill me with fatigue and soreness. I was more than fed up. I had worked so hard to gain a promotion and I was messing it up because my body was failing me.

He gave me a diagnosis of something physical: viral meningitis and prescribed anti-viral medication. I had far more symptoms than Dr Google listed for viral meningitis (headache, drowsiness, confusion, sensitivity to light, leg and back aches, bleeding, nausea, dizziness, abdominal pain, bladder and bowel pain) and the diagnosis was vague. But at least it was something. Something physical. Relieved I could finally reveal it wasn't just stress and I wasn't just being a crap teacher, I told my line manager. She snapped, 'Oh please, we've all had a virus before and we just get on with it!'

Well. Didn't that take the shine off! Exhausted, beaten down and scared of my body and brain's capacity to ruin everything for me, I was ready to give up. What was the point of anything anymore? Everything I loved, I lost because I wasn't capable of holding onto it. Everything I wanted, I found I couldn't do. And everything I won ended up being a bit of a curse. I was defeated.

I finished up my school day, got home and was about to fall into bed, but something made me get back up and take myself out for a walk.

Then came The Epiphany.

The Epiphany

It was a beautiful, warm, spring afternoon. I took a walk through the streets of Adelaide's beachside suburb of Glenelg. I was feeling contemplative while also having a complete existential crisis. I loved teaching, but clearly I wasn't cut out for it, if I was so stressed that my body was crashing.

I was so tired and hopeless. My whole body hurt and I felt like I was dying. I walked past a nursing home on a tree-lined street. The sun reflected off the 1960s facade and streamed through the large, velvet-curtained windows. I stopped to admire it. It really looked like a lovely place to spend the remaining days of one's twilight years.

I watched for a while as two people sat quietly in comfy armchairs gazing peacefully out the window (which in hindsight was probably a little creepy of me, but it was The Epiphany, so stay with me). *If that were me in that comfy chair in the final stage of my life,* I thought, *would I be happy with the decisions I'd made?* Remember, at this point, I felt like I was dying, so it was an entirely appropriate question to ask a person in their early thirties.

That's when it hit me. My whole life, I had wanted to be a writer (and a performer, and also to marry Leo DiCaprio but that ship had definitely sailed by then). Having missed so much school and after dropping out early (as well as having doctors tell me I was mentally unstable, and the fact I lacked confidence in general), I didn't think I was smart enough to ever be a writer. Particularly a magazine writer, which was my dream. But now that I was likely dying (I wasn't, but it felt that way so let's run with it), life was too short not to live as I desired. I was ready to start my life, at what felt like the end of my life. I made a rash, but excellent, decision to quit my permanent job and go back to uni to study journalism.

I resigned the next day. And I feel like this is where my life really began. I closed a door on a chapter that wasn't serving me and all the windows opened on the next chapter.

In 2012, I completed a year-long Postgraduate Diploma in Journalism while working in an outbound call centre, trying to sell a conservative newspaper to people who were unfortunate enough to answer their landlines. It was a wild experience and not my best choice of job, but it was a casual job in media that I could do while I was studying and which I could leave behind when I clocked off. There was no marking or extra-curricular commitments. I was very terrible at this job, but I had a chance to do some writing for the paper, which was an absolute dream and I adored that part of it.

By this stage, Matt and I had moved in together, along with his two young children Keeley and Niamh, who were two and four. So I was also an instant parent, which was so much fun. We did so much craft, singing, beach days, playing, learning *Frozen* by heart . . . I had never known such happiness.

Back when I was single and knee-deep in online dating, I had filtered out guys who had kids from the search function. I was desperate to have kids of my own, but I didn't want the complication of a partner who had children and an ex hanging around. But the filter doesn't work in real life and you can't help who you fall in love with. Besides, Matt's kids and ex-wife are excellent people, so I got lucky.

Those days after The Epiphany were wonderful and I was blissfully happy. Predictably, my job satisfaction in the outbound call centre wasn't high and I spent more time off the phone than on it, but it wasn't high stakes, like teaching.

I hated calling people to sell them something they didn't ask for and copping abuse I definitely deserved for calling them out of the blue and pitching a newspaper subscription to them at dinnertime. But it was one of the only jobs available in media, at a time where journo jobs were being slashed and no one was interested in taking on a journalism intern in her mid-thirties. (Like DiCaprio, they prefer them younger).

The call centre wasn't well paid and the sales work wasn't much fun (despite my colleagues being hilarious and lovely) but I persevered with it. Eventually (within a month) I was promoted (moved along) to another department, where I dealt with dispute resolution and customer complaints, which was a lot more stimulating.

Sadly, it was then I had my first pregnancy loss and had to take a significant amount of time off work due to extensive surgery and subsequent complications. With children to think of now, I needed to make decisions for the whole family. To avoid complete financial ruin and potential homelessness, I put on my rose-coloured glasses, packed up my dream of becoming a full-time writer and went back to teaching.

Teaching with endo – and a diagnosis at last!

I love being a teacher. I adore working with young people because they're so much fun; there's never a dull moment and every day is different. But it's physically and mentally demanding. In each classroom there are up to thirty young people whose lives are in your hands and who require attention at all times. When you're on yard duty, there can be up to a thousand young people under your duty of care.

As a high school teacher, each day's classes are usually in around seven different rooms across the school on various storeys. And each of those classes has a new set of students and its own culture, which requires preparation and consideration – each one of those teenagers is dealing with their own life stuff. At any one time, a high school teacher is educating about 150 students, having to know their names, business about their wellbeing, information about their academic progress, their parents' names and whether they are in the correct uniform. The intrinsic benefits are wonderful, but it's also exhausting even for the most able-bodied.

I took a couple of contracts in category two disadvantaged schools that were challenging, wonderful and exhausting – and which took a great deal of energy because many of the students were at risk, disengaged and had challenging behaviours.

In 2006, when I first started teaching, this was very much my bag. But eight years later, with a body now ravaged by undiagnosed disease and further damage from an ectopic, cornual pregnancy, I wasn't capable of breaking up fights, counselling kids through trauma and enduring the mental load of some really unfortunate situations I wish I could have saved the students from. (Like dangerous home situations, self-harm and risk-taking behaviours.)

I took a job at a high fee-paying private school. Those jobs are not necessarily easier – all kids have their own unique sets of issues and private schools involve more demands on your time – it was better resourced and there were very few challenging behaviours. This takes the pressure off. (It's a shame the schools that need the most funding and resourcing don't receive it, but that's a whole other book.)

While I was teaching at the High Fee-Paying School, I was finally diagnosed with endometriosis. I was thirty-six years old. It was such a relief, but I also had to take a lot of time to grieve. Grieve the diagnosis. Grieve the length of time I'd spent trying to treat my mental state, only to feel like a failure because I wasn't getting any better. And grieve because I wasn't ever going to get better: this disease is lifelong, chronic and incurable. That's a lot to take in. But it wasn't a death sentence and now it had a name. So at least I could stop thinking I was dying of an exotic tropical mystery illness. (I have no regrets about doing the epiphany journalism degree, though.)

Matt and I were trying to conceive and suffering loss after loss. I started taking sick days. That's something I never, ever did in teaching, because it's harder to write reliefs and plan for another teacher to cover your classes and yard duties than it is to just front up and do it yourself. But my condition became far worse after my endo ablation which, coupled with my pregnancy losses, caused me to take too much time off. I ran out of sick days.

I adored the students and I didn't want to disadvantage them, so I made the difficult decision to leave that job. I still dip in and out doing short contracts and relief teaching, because I miss it, but I have to resign myself to the fact that I will never teach full-time again, because I need to stop fighting my illness and, instead, work with it to find the best work and lifestyle for me and my family.

Full disclosure though: at the time I was teaching full-time, I was also working as a freelance journalist, a volunteer radio presenter, a part-time publicist and SEO copywriter – so there were good reasons for me being exhausted and overworked. I just had to make a choice about which one would be best for my body.

Career change: work flexibility being my own boss

Writing seemed like something I could do from home, with flexible hours and work environment. I applied for an enormous number of casual or part-time writer jobs but couldn't get an interview, because I was working as a teacher and didn't have enough commercial writing experience.

I realised if a job didn't exist that would suit my health and experiences, I had to make one. That's when I started my own company, Expressions Media, using my journalism and teaching qualifications to run workshops to teach people how to write for business, while also working as a writer, editor and proofreader. That has morphed into venue management, and work as a speaker, MC performer and comedian.

Now I can work at my own pace, on my own terms – and sometimes from bed. I recognise when my body is telling me to slow down and I will try to take my foot off the accelerator. Like when my pain starts to flare up and I need to work somewhere soft, comfortable and horizontal. Or when I can feel it's going to be a particularly bad month for brain fog or fatigue and I reschedule and restructure my work to suit. Or when my period/ovulation is causing me to vomit and faint and I need to be close to the bathroom. These are times when working for myself helps me to look after my illness. I'm also a morning person, so I often enjoy ploughing through work from 4am until midday and taking the rest of the day off, which doesn't suit a 9–5 work schedule.

When I was working in hospitality or even as a teacher, the option to work from home or to work flexibly was impossible. But I've been able to craft a position for myself where I can do that. It's not easy and when I don't work, I don't get paid, so that requires some planning and contingency. But overall, it's the best decision I've ever made. There's also the benefit of being my own boss and not being told what to do – because I'm a rebel and I prefer to stick it to the man. In my pyjamas. From my couch.

5 signs I need to slow down and work less:

1. My fatigue starts to slow me down to the point where I am forgetting things. (Like PIN codes, appointments, deadlines.)
2. My pain amps up and I am in muscle spasm. This means I need to be somewhere comfortable and safe. I can normally keep producing work, but I can't always do things in person.
3. People tell me I look tired or sick.
4. I'm getting snappy, irritable and impatient for no reason. (Hormones and pain are the reason.)

5. I start to feel like a giant sack of mouldy potatoes, which can only be fixed by a doona day and some time out to take the stress off my body.

Disclosing endo at work (Part 2): my story

Starting a business isn't easy. and it's certainly not a quick fix. I had a few clients I'd taken on while I was teaching, but I needed a bit of a buffer to keep me going, considering we had two kids and a couple of hungry cats in the house.

I took on a series of very part-time jobs to cover me during the times where work might dry up a little, like part-time media advisor for a politician, publicist at an arts festival, and education coordinator at an opera company. Each time, I was honest and told my boss upfront I have endometriosis and I might need to occasionally work from home, but I would always be available via phone and email and the tasks would always get done. From state parliament to large arts organisations, the response differed. But it was largely positive and people were generally accommodating.

My politician boss, Tammy, was excellent about it, because she knew the work would be done and she knew she could contact me via phone or message. With some managers, it took some explaining. One boss wondered why I wanted flexible work conditions for a bad breath condition and we laughed for about an hour when I explained the difference between halitosis and endometriosis.

But it was the micromanagers who really found it difficult to process. You know who I'm talking about, right? The ones who want everything in a spreadsheet in shared folders, so they can watch what you're doing in real time and ask why you didn't fill in cell F35 in a timely manner. The ones who will call with a seemingly innocuous question that ends up an interrogation about what your office buddy has been up to, or asking you to talk through every single task on your to-do list. (And they'll then give you another, bigger pile of work to do.) The ones who fucking love a meeting that could have been a fucking email!

Sorry.

No, I'm not.

I took on a very part-time job in an organisation that I thought would be pleasant and engaging. And I had a really charismatic manager who seemed super understanding in the interview, when I told her I would largely be okay managing my illness, but some days I would need to work from home. I explained that my head was fine for thinking, my hands can type and my face can take calls, but my pain from my waist down would sometimes make sitting at a desk uncomfortable. At these times, I'd need to lie down, change location, elevate my legs to take the weight off my pelvis, or do whatever else would make me comfortable and more efficient. I said I would need to be close to a bathroom lest I vomit, and soft furnishings in case I faint.

She seemed totally cool with that and added a clause in my contract that said I was required to spend one day of a two-day per week job in the office, but the other day could be anywhere. It was a remarkably fair compromise, I thought. And, just as I had informed her, I was largely okay and didn't need to work from home until about six months into the job, when I had a pain flare-up and let her know I was going to use my work-from-home clause that day.

She said, 'Nope, if you're sick, you're sick. Take a sick day.'

I thought we had a good relationship, so I reminded her that being sick and being chronically ill were different. I was quite okay to work: I just needed to be in my own space to do it. She said, 'If you're okay to work, then you're okay to come in' and hung up on me.

So I went into work, spent most of the day sweating from the pain and the other part of the day trying to get comfortable on an upright swivel chair. Of course, she also called a meeting to discuss the spreadsheet and cell F35. This boss, who I thought was chill and understanding, was equally sympathetic (ie. not at all) about my pregnancy losses. She gave me a hard time when I had my second ectopic pregnancy by telling me I'd let the team down with my absence – just in case I wasn't feeling bad enough.

Endo at work: other people's stories

Other people I've spoken to have had varied responses to their disclosure of their illness, but I think we should be able to share with our bosses what we need – and they should be accommodating with reasonable requests for making a workplace accessible.

Gem works in retail and has had both positive and negative experiences with her employers. In her current job at a baby goods store, her boss is accommodating, understanding and offers flexibility for her working conditions. But it hasn't always been like that in her career, especially when she worked in the adult industry.

'I've had so many issues with sick days because of bosses who don't understand endometriosis and don't want to. I have done shifts with wheat bags and heat packs strapped to me while being accused of slacking off because I go to the toilet too much,' she says.

'With all my gut troubles around my cycle I have definitely pooped myself at work.'

I queried whether the adult industry might have been better equipped to deal with issues of the uterus, given that bodies are their specialty, but Gem set me straight.

'Oh no, no, no,' she laughs. 'It's still a very male-driven industry, with way less understanding of women's health issues than other industries. The adult retail industry is just like any other retail really, except the bosses just have their fingers in shadier pies.'

And speaking of the adult industry, sex worker Mona has had to pack up her business – not because of bad bosses, but because her pelvic pain has become too unbearable to continue working. I have known Mona for many years. She has always had such enthusiasm for her industry and loves her work, but she is having to plan for a career change because the painful sex is debilitating and her flare-ups are limiting her opportunities to see clients.

'I just can't do it anymore. The sex wasn't really an issue up until recently where my periods have just become extremely painful. I mean, my periods have always been ridiculously painful but last year the cramps just dropped me to my knees,' she says. 'And now sex hurts during and after. I can't even have an orgasm because it hurts too much. Well, I can, but I get severe cramps afterwards and it's almost not worth it. Almost.'

We laugh about that, because we both know she'd give it a crack anyway. But it's not just the pain that affects business. Mona has been dealing with gut issues that are can be a very annoying and unpleasant symptom of endo.

'One of the symptoms I wasn't aware of was nausea. And I do trips to Mount Gambier (the traditional lands of the Boadik People) where I'm booked out. One trip, I had a client on the second night I was there. I felt nauseous. I told him I wasn't feeling very well and within five minutes I was running to the toilet and vomiting. Luckily, he was a regular and was lovely about it,' she says. 'I thought it was the truck-stop fast food until I realised it was the pain doing it.'

For now, Mona is still seeing some clients, but her work has been limited by her illness and she is now transitioning into administrative work to keep herself financially afloat. She is making accommodations so she can still perform some tasks, but there are some bookings she just can't accept anymore.

'Basically doggie style is a no-go and, if I have anyone that's above average in (penis) size, I end up in pain or bleeding or both,' she says. 'With all my clients now, I'm always on top so I'm in control of the pace and depth. And I use other methods to make it over quicker, whether that's dirty talk, or extending foreplay. Luckily, I've always run my bookings where I start off with a striptease for that very reason. So, you get them all worked up and then the actual business end of it is over a lot quicker.

'I've got two regular clients, they're both disabled, and they're lovely. They book me for extended or overnight bookings and I'm keeping them, but I've lost so much money having to drop work. And I can't tell the clients. One of my regulars who I see every week is a great guy: books half an hour; he's in and out on time every week without fail. But what do I tell him? He's not entitled to my personal information.'

My career space is not as physical as Mona's, but now that I understand my strengths and limitations, I try to be completely honest with people so they know where I'm at. But it always catches me off guard when someone is inflexible or not inclusive.

Endo-friendly (and unfriendly) workplaces

Thankfully, most bosses are absolutely cool with it; most of the time they know someone with endo. But I made a promise that if they freak out or refuse to accommodate me and my condition, they're not people I want to work with. If they haven't listened, they never will. That's not a culture I'm interested in being part of.

I know I always get the work done and I perform to a very high standard – but sometimes, I will need to do that from the safety of my home. When I employ contractors or host interns, I am always flexible with when, where and how they work. As long as the work comes in and they're around at our agreed times, I am happy for them to work however it suits them.

A shout-out here to the excellent bosses and workplaces out there who are doing the right things to be inclusive, accepting, and help people with endo to have a good quality of life, preserving their right to work. This accessibility and inclusivity should work: ethically, legally and morally.

Victoria University are one of the good ones, says provisional Masters by Research candidate Michelle Gissara. She is researching *Ngarnga Nanggit ('Wisdom of the Elders'): An Intergenerational*

Oral History of the Koori Courts in Victoria under a fully funded scholarship, with accommodations for her disability and chronic illness.

'The uni classifies both endometriosis and fibromyalgia as chronic illness and disability, so I have accessibility plans and I am able to get extensions for assignments if I need them,' she says. 'I had different provisions for exams to be able to stop and go to the toilet and things like that, which with endo, is sometimes urgent. Especially having lesions on the bladder and bowels.'

Michelle's workplace deserves a shout-out for being inclusive and excellent. However, Linda's boss gets a big thumbs down from me. Linda joined the armed forces when she was nineteen. She was referred to a gynae in the military and diagnosed with endo on her twenty-first birthday. Being in that male-dominated environment in the '90s, where there was a need to be 'tough', was difficult for this brave and resilient woman who was working in engineering.

'It was horrible, to be honest. It was good as far as getting the best possible treatment, because we got the best surgeons and I got access to Zoladex [a hormonal implant that can be used to treat symptoms of endometriosis] when that was first released – which was really expensive and not on the PBS at the time,' she says. 'But as far as how you were treated by your peers, it was just appalling. You were a malingerer. You were a sook. You needed to have a cup of concrete,' she says.

'There was only about one girl to one hundred men and they were just vile. My first laparoscopy was on my twenty-first birthday and I had to get up and go back to work the next day and march with everybody. I was basically told to suck it up.'

Wow. That is brutal. Luckily Linda is now working in a job she loves, helping to place foster children with long-term families. And there's no marching, which is good.

Supporting workers with endometriosis in the workplace

In 2018, as part of the National Action Plan for Endometriosis, the 'Supporting workers with endometriosis in the workplace' information sheet was created to help employers increase awareness of how common and serious endo is, its impact on workers and how that affects workplace health and safety. It instructs employers that:

> Informing yourself about endometriosis can lead to better workplace outcomes. You will be prepared to support workers affected by endometriosis if you have a good understanding of the disease and the reasonable steps that you can take to help workers manage their symptoms. Women, girls and other individuals with endometriosis say that having the disease recognised and acknowledged by people around them, such as their managers, can positively influence their experience.[10]

It's a great resource to have on hand if you are not comfortable explaining your condition to your employer and you need a bit of back-up, like Astrid needed when she worked as a receptionist and she wasn't permitted to go home sick after being struck down with an endo flare.

'I was in so much pain that I was sweating,' she says. 'They wouldn't let me leave early and I had no painkillers, so I forced my belly against the desk and corseted myself against the desk rim as pain relief.'

Not only would this have been humiliating: it's also dangerous to have someone in that much pain in the office using a desk as a method of pain control. Where are the overbearing occupational health and safety officers with their clipboards and hard hats when you actually need them? Astrid was also in a position where she was

10   https://www.safeworkaustralia.gov.au/doc/supporting-workers-endometriosis-workplace

greeting clients and visitors as they came in the door, so keeping her at work in pain and not allowing her to go home to tend to her symptoms really benefited no one.

But it's not all bad news. Kylie Maslen, author of *Show Me Where it Hurts*[11] has endeavoured to create positive work experiences, despite having debilitating invisible illnesses, such as polycystic ovarian syndrome, endometriosis, bipolar disorder and chronic pelvic pain. Kylie works with arts organisations to produce festivals and events, which can involve administrative work and a lot of physically demanding, on-site work. But she has found a way to make it work so she can still do a job she loves without it ruining her health. It wasn't always like that, though, and it took a crisis point to change the way she was approaching work and her illnesses.

'In 2017, the chronic pain had got to a point where I began to identify as disabled; it was that kind of turning point where I couldn't work full-time anymore, it was having a real impact on my day-to-day life. I was thirty-five,' she says.

'It wasn't until that really bad flare-up that I actually kind of stopped to think about how work was affecting my health,' she says.

Listening to Kylie, who I adore and admire, I have had another 'aha!' moment. I have always prioritised and catastrophised how my health was affecting my work, rather than how the work was affecting my health. But the way Kylie says it makes much more sense – and was actually the catalyst for me making changes to the way I prioritise health and work. Some of the healthiest decisions I made about my work-life balance were after this conversation with her.

'It took getting to a real crisis point for me to make changes,' she says. 'I was working as an events producer through freelance jobs back-to-back for years. And it's the kind of job that is high adrenaline.

---

11   Maslen, Kylie, 'Show Me Where It Hurts', Text Publishing, Australia, 2020

'And it's very rewarding, but it's incredibly taxing. I worked primarily in arts festivals, and I thought, *I'm not going to be able to work a festival again*, but my employers said, *Look, we recognise that this is just going to be too much, but we really want to keep you on, so how about we restructure it? How many days do you feel capable of doing? We can get you to do the stuff that you really specialise in and get other people to do the stuff that is a bit more widespread.*'

Living in Melbourne at the time, Kylie wanted to move home to Adelaide to be closer to her support network. Her employers happily accepted the relocation so she could continue working with them while prioritising her health.

'Out of complete chance, two of the directors had moved back to Adelaide earlier that year and set up an office here, and so they said, *We see that you really need to be with your family at the moment and we want to accommodate that,*' she says.

'But, to be perfectly honest, it took being suicidal to get to this point where that shift really needed to happen. The past few years have been really challenging while I've been going through my bipolar diagnosis and finding the right med balance. They've been so understanding, even though they've had no experience with this before.'

Having created a safe space and a support team, Kylie has been able to carve out a career where she can work in the fields she loves in a way that benefits her and her employers.

'It's really hard, I'm not going to lie about that, but there are now systems in place for when shit goes bad, basically. And that help and those systems have also been communicated in a way that makes sense to me. There are step-by-step plans in place,' she says.

Communication has been the key to Kylie's relationship with her employers, which has made it possible for her to continue working in a way that isn't detrimental to her health and wellbeing.

'It's a small company, but also just incredible people who really look after their staff, and they've really made me feel like family, during some really shit times. I'm transparent with them about what's going on, and I certainly tell them more than I would have told other employers over the years, undoubtedly because the more I tell them what's happening, the more that they can plan around it, and therefore be able to keep me on,' she says. 'And they're really transparent with me about what they need to know and what they're thinking in terms of what projects they might need to reassign me from or to.'

Negotiating positive change: my story

Hearing this motivates me to be better at communicating with people. In the past, I would rather set myself on fire than tell someone I need more time for a project, because I have so much shame attached to asking for help. Kylie's story stirs something in me.

I have made some positive changes, like choosing only to work on projects and clients that align with my values and who are respectful of my time and wellbeing. I am now honest with people about the times I am sick and how that will affect my work output. As I get older, I am becoming less physically able, but I'm becoming better at communicating with people.

I took on a client with whom I called a meeting to discuss their needs and how we can work together, ready to make my big step into communicating my needs and work methods. I talked about how we could complement each other. I explained I don't work Thursdays because I'm with my foster son all day. I told them I prefer email communication because then I have a paper trail, which works better for when my brain fog causes me to forget things. And I said I needed them to submit a briefing sheet with deadlines so I could prioritise tasks and complete things in a timely manner for them.

I was pretty chuffed about my big, grown-up approach and was high-fiving myself. Until Thursday came and I received eight phone calls, three text messages, four urgent emails and a partridge in a pear tree. Not only had they ignored my boundaries: they weren't respecting my time. So I completed their tasks the next day and respectfully ended the working relationship.

They needed someone who could be on-call and always available and that's not me. But someone else will do a stellar job for them. In the past I would have beaten myself up over that and felt like it was a personal failure. But it's not. It's just not a compatible working relationship. And that's okay.

Choosing to only take on things that feel right has been a privilege, but it's also been self-care. My mate, fellow freelancer and co-working buddy Peta says, 'If it's not a hell yeah, it's a no'. I take that into everything I do now. If I don't feel completely positive about a situation, I don't get involved with it, because I don't have the mental or physical bandwidth to deal with it and then clean up the aftermath. Here's a callback to earlier, when I told you this excellent advice from a friend: 'I have never once regretted saying no to doing something I didn't feel well enough to do, but I have always regretted saying yes.'

It's taken a long time to prioritise my physical and mental health, but I'm glad I am now and it's working very well for me. I am choosing better projects that have more successful outcomes – and I am happier and less stressed. If you take on every little thing because you think people will be unhappy if you don't, you need to remember they are more unhappy if you take it on and can't commit to it because you've spread yourself too thin.

My FOMO (fear of missing out) is significant, so I hate saying no to things. But I am learning to see my limitations and know the opportunity will come up again if it's right. But it's not beneficial to either party if I agree to do something and then can't deliver. I have made many mistakes by doing this and I don't want to do it anymore. I have ended up in some very difficult situations simply by taking on more than I can handle and not being able to find my way out or communicate what I need to help me.

What not to do in the workplace (for employers)

I have been at the point of being suicidal when I've felt overwhelmed, unable to communicate, and trying to stay afloat, like the chronic people pleaser I am. Communication, for me, feels overwhelming when I'm at my worst.

I suffered three pregnancy losses in as many months in the admin job I mentioned earlier (remember the one where the boss wouldn't let me work from home even though it was in my contract?). I worked so hard throughout those losses, even when I was in hospital with my second ectopic pregnancy (when the embryo implants in the tube and is not viable). After the ectopic was blasted with Methotrexate (a medicine often used in chemotherapy, which is prescribed in some ectopic pregnancies to stop the rapid growth of cells), I had to go back to hospital every day to have blood tests to check the hormones were settling and getting back to base. I would do it at the start or end of my workday so I didn't let the team down. But the trauma and exhaustion caught up with me after a couple of weeks and I started making mistakes.

Rather than reach out and say, 'Hey, what do you need? How can we help? We've noticed that you've dropped the ball on some things', the boss dragged me into the office and raked me over the coals, raising her voice with the door open so everyone could hear. I was at my lowest of lows. I was on my tenth pregnancy loss in total and three of those had been in very quick succession. I already felt completely hopeless and profoundly sad. The grief was all-consuming. But this was the nail in the coffin. I walked out of her office, shaking. I'd let everyone down. I was a failure. I couldn't keep a pregnancy, I couldn't do my job, I couldn't get well. I couldn't do anything.

I made up my mind to end my life that night.

I packed up my desk so I didn't leave a mess. I planned to go home, clean the house and do the laundry so my family wouldn't have to worry about it. And then I was going to end my life.

But on my way out the door, a colleague gently stepped out of her office, stood in my way and stopped me. She sat me down and held my hand. She'd heard the dressing-down I received from the boss and she knew I'd been in and out of hospital over the past six weeks. *We can fix this,* she said. *We can turn this around. I want to help you. I've got you.* I said nothing. I just started to cry. And I couldn't stop crying. I cried like a tiny baby: sobbing, purging, wailing, releasing all the hurt, grief, loss, anger and hopelessness. She held me. I crumbled.

We did turn it around. With her help, I fixed the couple of mistakes I made, caught up on the things I needed to complete and then I resigned from the job. No job is worth dying over. I will forever be grateful to her for saving my life that day.

Communication works both ways. I should have asked for help and my employer should have told me they were concerned about me and asked if I needed help. Even if we didn't turn it around, and I didn't finish those jobs or fix those mistakes, the world wouldn't have ended and the crimes I'd committed were not punishable by death. But I was so scared to ask for help that I was willing to be beaten by a situation that, in hindsight – while stressful and horrible – was not so bad I needed to walk away from everything and everyone I love.

Fighting guilt and asking for support

'I completely understand the fear of, *Will it cost me this opportunity at work?* But not talking about what's going on doesn't benefit anyone,' Kylie Maslen says. 'A lot of people still don't understand what endometriosis is, let alone what it looks and feels like. So, as much as it sucks that the onus is still primarily on the person in pain to at least instigate the conversation, being open about your circumstances with the people in your life – and that includes employers as well as your support network and family – gives people an understanding of what's going on, so that they can help you.'

Sage advice. And Syl from EndoActive agrees, saying while it's perfectly normal to feel bad about taking a break or being unable to do things, the guilt can consume you, and communication always clears the path.

'It's really easy to beat yourself up, feel guilty about all the things that you're not achieving and can't achieve. And then it just gives you really bad anxiety. I used to get anxious that everyone was talking about me and saying I'm a flake and I'm not showing up to this or that. And as I've gone on and developed the EndoActive community, I will still sometimes be inactive on social media and I have this constant voice in the back of my head telling me off, telling me I'm a bad person, I'm a failure, I'm a fuck-up, for not doing it,' she says.

'And a few times I have reached out to our community and said, *Hey guys, I'm really sorry I haven't been active on here. I'm needing to take a break for either physical health or mental health or have other work on* and they always respond with, *You don't need to tell us that. You shouldn't need to ask permission to take a break. We get it better than anyone else does.* But it's probably a bit harder for people who don't have a chronic illness to understand that.'

Donna from Endometriosis Australia echoes the guilt sentiment and the need to be productive when you can. I get it: I like to try to make hay while the sun shines and get as much done as I can before the pain or brain fog strikes again.

'My biggest thing is that I feel guilty if I'm not productive,' says Donna. 'Even recovering from surgeries, I had to have something to tick off the list and say, *look what I did!* So, I crocheted a blanket. It took years, but it was in between the surgeries and that recovery phase. Another thing was sorting through tax receipts, filling that need to be productive and contributing. I still want to feel that I've got value. I just don't want the disease to take that away from who I am.'

There will always be managers who will discriminate, for any illness or disability. By law, they're not actually allowed to. But regardless of whether you're an employee, employer, CEO, trainee, or stay-at-home parent, work can have an impact on your chronic condition. So it's important to take a break, manage your time and communicate.

QENDO's Jess Taylor is an absolute dynamo. She is constantly working and always creating a new project or way to help or inspire people with endo – while managing her full-time work duties, commitments to the endo community and being a parent. In fact, she never seems to stop.

'I think that there's a level of being scared that if we stop, if we don't push through, if we get off this merry-go-round, we won't know how to live,' she says. 'But if you do, you will actually achieve more. It can be such a mental load to have all this stuff to think about all the time. But I have achieved so much when I've stepped off every once in a while.'

If there's one thing the Covid-19 pandemic taught us, it's that it's possible – and practical – to work from home. (Though of course, not in all jobs – for example, retail, hospitality or factory work.) Many occupations have now proven to be just as effectively and efficiently done when worked remotely. Like all of those fucking meetings that could have been a fucking email.

With any luck, this will open up a whole new world for people with chronic illness, which will improve our physical and mental health, and give us a fighting chance to live to our full potential.

Because not all jobs can be performed at home, it's important to communicate your needs to your employer and let them know it's a health and safety requirement to accommodate reasonable requests.

6 tips for communicating with your boss:

1. Give them the 'Supporting workers with endometriosis in the workplace' information sheet and have a conversation about what that means for you. Follow up in writing about what was discussed so you have a record of it.

2. Your health is important. This is the only body you've got, so treat it well and have others do the same. Consider the impact your work has on your health, not the other way around.

3. If your colleagues don't understand your illness, they might catastrophise it or minimise it. Having a simple definition prepared can help to explain it. Something like, *Endo is a chronic, incurable illness where tissue that's like the lining of the uterus grows in other places causing inflammation and sometimes our organs stick together which is very painful.* This works because sometimes when you mention periods to people, they dismiss them with *oh it's just period pain* or they get grossed out and stop listening.

4. Talk to your employer about flexible work situations where possible. Whether that's working from home or completing tasks where you can sit down for a bit or limit physical labour like lifting or bending.

5. Be upfront about your illness. Explain that it won't always affect you, but when it does, you may need some time out.

6. I don't take any bullshit from people who want to treat me like I'm making things up or exaggerating for effect. I have put up with more than enough of that rubbish and I'm done with it. I have an illness and, just like sufferers of diabetes, asthma, or any other affliction, I deserve support, understanding, respect and consideration. And so do you.

9

Partners in Pain

endo allies and supporting spouses

Being a partner of someone with a chronic illness is a challenge. I take my hat off to anyone who is a spouse, parent, bestie or support person for a chronically ill patient. Seriously, I can barely handle living with myself. I have no idea how you folks do it.

When I was single and lived alone, I didn't know I had endo. Pre-diagnosis, I was often unwell and would cancel plans, not turn up to things or struggle through events or occasions miserable and in pain. My family sometimes assumed I was drunk or hungover, because I was working in bars at the time. Don't get me wrong: sometimes I *did* have a belting hangover, or was spending the day in bed with one of my poor choices. But more often, it was because I worked three jobs at a time to put myself through uni, and on my days off I was exhausted or scrambling to get essays in.

I was also embarrassed that I was physically ill from stress and worry (as diagnosed by my GPs) because I have a solid work ethic inherited from my father, who rarely took a sickie and worked about twenty hours a day. It was humiliating to be cancelling family events due to things like panic attacks in the video store.

These days, I try to listen to my body when it tells me to stop – which has meant I'm ill far less often than I otherwise would be. My respiratory system is not good and never has been. I used to thrash myself by working long hours at multiple jobs until my immune system would crash and I'd end up with a flu, which would turn into something worse, like tonsillitis or pneumonia. This meant that when I had time off, I would figuratively hit a wall and be no good to anyone. So, I was often quite an unreliable friend or family member. I loved people like mad, but bailed on things with about the same amount of enthusiasm.

In pre-diagnosis relationships (I've had two husbands, three fiancés, a couple of girlfriends and quite a few boyfriends), I was probably very hard work. Especially since I was often in pain, sometimes unwell and would faint and vomit due to pain or ovulation (which I did not connect the dots on at the time, on account of my life being too hectic and never knowing what day it was, so I never tracked my cycle until iPhones became a thing). I couldn't explain my lethargy or pain, so it was a source of conflict in many relationships. Once, on a date, I fainted during a romantic walk down by a creek. *Must be a panic attack,* I explained to partner at the time, who urged me to see a psychologist.

I booked in to see a psych, who was an affable, older man who reminded me of my beloved, late grandfather. I immediately felt at home in his presence . . . until he fixed his eyes on me, leaned in and said seriously and steadily, 'Libby, you are fainting because you are holding your breath'. He went on, and I actually find myself laughing aloud as I write this, 'You are behaving like a toddler who throws a tantrum to get their own way and holds their breath until they turn blue and pass out.'

He had fancy certificates on the wall and a water feature in the foyer, so I took his word as law. But the next time I felt faint, I noticed I was alone (so there was no one around to perform for) and I was definitely breathing, so that logic was flawed. But I paid him $400 for this absolute pearl of a story to tell you. Bargain.

Matt and me: period and pain talk is not taboo in our house

I got my endo diagnosis while I was with my (second) husband,

Matt. He is sweet, funny, talented, endlessly patient, creative and clever. He's the best person I know. Matt and I make a good team. We work together, make theatre shows together and we run programs and workshops together. We also parent three children together.

We've spoken with our two girls about periods as soon as it was age appropriate to do so, because we wanted to make sure they were prepared. Matt chats about periods with us, too: we don't feel it should just be something that people assigned female at birth should deal with. It's not a taboo subject in our house. It's a big, natural part of our lives.

It was always important to us that our daughters weren't scared of periods – and that they knew that, just because my pain and symptoms are shitty, it didn't mean theirs would be. But just in case, we looked at ways they might combat period cramps through easy pelvic stretches, medications that block prostaglandins and heat packs. They are such clever and switched-on girls and I am the luckiest person to be their stepmother. They have processed the information really well and have a good knowledge of menstrual health, which is normalised in our home.

Pain is not normalised in our home.

We now have a little boy in our family who came to live with us while I was writing this book. We intend to be just as open and honest with him about menstrual health, so he can be an excellent advocate, too.

There are many ways to help someone with chronic illness, but it's not easy. So if you are a partner, you need to be one hundred per cent in. Your partner with endo doesn't have the luxury of dipping in and out, so you can't either. Having said that, it's a good idea to set boundaries and let your partner know your capacity to be there and what you are willing to take on – otherwise things can get messy and people can get hurt.

Sarah and Carla: 'part and parcel of our life'

Dr Sarah Van Der Wal, a gynaecologist and obstetrician living with endo, has total support at home from their partner Carla, which makes living with the condition so much easier, particularly with their demanding job.

'Sometimes I'll come home and I'll be absolutely cactus, and, I'll just be like, *I can't do the dishes tonight* and she'll say, *Yeah, whatever. Don't do the dishes.* I'll flop into bed exhausted, and say, *I'm having an endo flare.* And usually, I just get a hug and a *goodnight, off you go*, and she'll give me painkillers if I need them,' Sarah says.

'We've been together for nineteen years, since I was in early med school. It's just really part and parcel of our life. This is just what she does. We're pretty good with each other in general, I like to think.'

Claire and Anthony: 'He makes it possible for me to live'

Claire's husband Anthony is a huge support to her. Claire's chronic pain condition is severe and because her job as a theatre-maker, director and drama teacher is quite physical, she more than appreciates the support she receives from him.

'He makes it possible for me to live. He does so much for me. He brings me my heat packs. He runs my baths. He drives me places. He cooks dinner. He cleans up. He gets up early so that I don't have to. He does stuff like vacuuming that I can't do. He will always meet me after work so that I can stop pretending. And, well, he believes me,' she says.

Claire was diagnosed twenty-six years after her symptoms first presented. She tries to find the best ways to live as comfortably as she can. She and Anthony have gone through a lot together to learn about the illness and work out strategies to survive it.

'I think I'm probably different now. I think maybe my personality has changed. I was always a grumpy person. He knew that from the very second we met,' Claire laughs. 'But now I think that I get down for longer. And I think I got sick of talking about it all out loud. So now I internalise things a lot more. So, he just has to put up with me being silent for long periods of time and then he knows something's wrong. I'm working on it with my therapist. She focuses on getting deep into my brain to try to see what's connected to pain and find out whether we can fix my brain to hopefully stop it from firing all of its nerve endings all the time. I find her really helpful.'

For Anthony, life has changed as a result of Claire's illness, but he has adapted and changed with it, because he adores her. It's 2020 and I'm speaking with the couple via video call with Matt. We both order UberEats at the same time so we can have dinner together, because it's the only way we can catch up in a pandemic.

'Life can be difficult now,' Anthony says. 'I don't mean difficult in a bad way. I think it brings a certain level of uncertainty to our lives. Prior to the diagnosis, we were able to properly plan a lot more, or plan ahead – in terms of a weekend or our lives. Whereas I think now, we pretty much live day-to-day a lot more. There are events we try to attend, so we say, *Okay, well, this is coming up. How are you going to deal with this situation? And what drugs do we have available to get you through this day?*

'But, in a positive way we are much more flexible now, because we go, *Okay, how are you feeling? What can you get through? Maybe we need to go to bed on this night because you were so exhausted physically by the day.* It has been a reasonably long transitional journey. About four years ago, when it became really bad for her, was quite difficult in both our lives, just trying to adjust to that new routine.

'Now we have gone through that period of adjustment and we both know what to expect and are able to better track the pain cycle, we can say, *Okay, we know you might have a good (I use that phrase loosely), week here and then a really bad week here, depending on what's happening with your body at the time.* And we try to take advantage of that a bit more as well.'

'You're also really good at knowing when I shouldn't do things,' Claire laughs. 'And then I do them anyway and then you're like, *I thought that might not have been the best idea because you're about to get your period.*'

But Anthony's kindness, generosity and patience doesn't extend to Claire's health practitioners, who haven't been able to offer as much support as the couple would have liked.

'It's completely undermined the little faith I previously had in the medical system. I thought, *Okay, they've given their diagnosis now. This is what it is. I'm sure we'll be able to work to something that means she can live a normal life.* And essentially there's very little they can do. And so, you're like, *Oh great, you've seen a thousand doctors and none of them have offered anything to improve your quality of life to a great degree.*'

Despite all that, Claire and Anthony have battled through to find their relationship is stronger and more resilient as a result of their hardships.

'Having to help Claire through her pain, just knowing that my presence is sometimes required, even if there are no words required, has given a closer bond as a couple,' Anthony says.

And if he were to offer advice to other partners of people with endo?

'The first thing I would say is to believe what your partner is saying – unlike the medical profession – and just listen and empathise. Don't put pressure on them to talk about how they're feeling if they don't want to talk at that particular time. Just be supportive. Know that there will possibly never be a cure, and treatments may not work, but just be there to help them through that process. Help your partner recognise their limits, but also help them strive to overachieve,' he says.

'And get ready for less sex,' Claire interjects.

Penetrative sex, pelvic physio and OhNuts

It is true that penetrative intercourse can cause pain for people with endometriosis. Not everyone. But for some, it can be really difficult. Finding a pelvic physio can be helpful to relax those muscles, but also to find out where the muscle tightness is and what exercises and treatments you can do to ease that. There are dilators that come in a range of sizes that will work to restore vaginal capacity, to expand the area and help with elasticity to the tissues, which can help make penetrative sex more comfortable. If tampons are difficult to use, a pelvic physio can help with that as well.

It's funny – and I always laugh about this with fellow endo patients – but it is a myth that all women love enormous dicks and sex that goes for hours. Trust me, whoever started those rumours probably didn't have endometriosis (no judgment if you have endo and love a big one that goes forever). But if you are in a situation where you have a partner who has a large penis and penetrative sex is painful, you can get soft, silicone rings called OhNuts (they look like doughnuts) that go on the base of penis. OhNuts shorten the depth of penetration for the endo patient and retain the pleasure for the penis-owner. They are reusable and last a long time. There are other brands on the market as well.

'My boyfriend and I bought a set of OhNuts and it has saved our sex life,' Chrissy (twenty-five) says. 'I was so scared of sex and he was always so scared of hurting me, but after we bought the rings, we have been so much more relaxed about it and sex is fun again. I was so worried I'd hate sex forever, and it's taken me a while to feel completely safe again – also, Dylan was very reluctant to use them at first but when he did, he said he couldn't tell the difference between me and the rings when we lubed them up! It's made a big difference for us.'

Not every endo patient will have trouble with sex, but it's something to consider when supporting someone with the disease, or when you start dating them. Endo patients will need to do things at their own pace. Also, you'll need to learn to recognise the difference between noises of passion and noises of pain, which can be subtle, but is important.

Unfortunately, due to circumstances beyond our control (ie. the patriarchy), some people assigned female at birth who are in relationships with men have been conditioned to stay quiet if they are uncomfortable during sex, so as not to ruin the mood. But honestly, it's not worth the pain and you are worth more than that. So, speak up if it's hurting! And if you are the partner, listen and observe and know when they're not into it (this advice can also apply to every area of life where consent is involved).

Navigating pain and intimacy

Supporting someone with a pain condition means learning a whole new language of recognising noises, facial expressions and movements. But if a partner isn't willing to do that, it can have a major impact on the person with the illness. Carla's partner left because he refused to understand why she didn't want to have sex every day.

'In the beginning of our relationship, we had stacks of great sex, but then as I got older and my endo got worse, sex just became uncomfortable. I would worry about it, which made me tense, and then it was awkward because it just didn't work. Then I'd cry and he'd get mad and we'd fight and do it all again the next day,' she says. 'Honestly, it was a relief when he left, but it's put me off being in an intimate relationship for a long while, if ever.'

I know in many of my relationships (quick refresher: two husbands, three fiancés, a couple of girlfriends and quite a few boyfriends), the intimacy has been a problem for me. And up until my diagnosis, I would just grin and bear it. Sometimes literally. I am a very sensual, affectionate and physical person and at the time, I didn't know why I was so uncomfortable. I didn't ever want to ruin a moment, nor did I want my partners to think I didn't want them, so I would go along with sex even when it was hurting or I

153

didn't feel up to it. This ended up being quite traumatic on many occasions. I don't recommend it. I do highly recommend knowing your limits and not pushing them, having clear communication and absolutely saying no if you don't want it. Partners must respect that. Sex is only good if everyone is into it.

Michelle has struggled with intimacy in her relationships due to pain. Even though she's now in a strong and loving partnership, intimacy still offers some real challenges.

'My main endo pain is with sex and bowel pain. I do have abnormal pain leading up to and during my period for many days, but that wasn't as much of a red flag as the deep, stabbing pain with sexual intercourse and pain going to the toilet. This type of pain has mostly affected my intimate relationships,' she says.

'Experiencing stabbing pain with penetrative intercourse has resulted in me suffering major anxiety around being intimate. Even the thought of kissing, leading to touching, leading to sex makes me recoil. Luckily, I have an extremely understanding partner who is very supportive and we try lots of different ways to be intimate and communicate very openly. But it is a daily struggle to be intimate when I know the pain is coming. This pain has affected my mental health in many ways. I have been working with a pain psychologist and sex therapist as well as a pelvic floor physiotherapist, but it is a long road and my pain is still present post-laparoscopy.'

Managing my limits

In my relationship with Matt, we have had to make room for this illness by changing a lot of things. But that's been a dream come true for me, because I'd always wanted to live better and within my limits. I've always had endo: I just didn't have the tools to deal with it or a name for it.

I've changed my attitude, adjusted my self-talk and worked on my acceptance and self-forgiveness. But I've also changed how much I do, cut down on my overcommitting and am making choices that benefit me, Matt and the kids, and the business. Because those are the things that matter to me. It's made me change my priorities and stop being such a chronic people pleaser, which I've been my whole life.

Physically, I've changed the way I approach intimacy by having boundaries. Another physical change I've made is my shoes. It's been the best decision. I don't wear heels at all, ever. I only wear flats now and it has changed my whole world. Now I don't get three days of shooting pain up my legs, back and rectum after a night in stilettos, because my pelvis is in spasm from tottering around on spikes. I buy gorgeous flatties and it more than halves my pain when I go out. I know there are people who are incredibly empowered by wearing heels – and if it makes you feel good, do it. (Just put in place a pain management plan for when you climb off them, so you can keep rocking them.)

And I use a walking stick when I need one – especially if I am at an event where I need to do a lot of standing and not enough chairs are available. I've also bought an electric bike, which is super fun and makes zipping around the city easier and more efficient – and means I don't have to walk too far on high pain days, but I can still get a bit of exercise.

Matt's story: a partner's perspective

I've talked a lot about me. What's it like for Matt? Let's hear him talk about me! I interviewed my husband while he was enjoying a glass of red wine in front of a roaring fire in Cudlee Creek in the Adelaide Hills (the lands of the Peramangk and Kaurna peoples). Fun story: When Matt told my stepdaughters he was taking me to Cudlee Creek they thought it was a euphemism for sex and were completely grossed out, until we explained through tears of laughter that it was a self-imposed writer's retreat getaway. Anyway, I digress.

During this interview, Matt is laying on a cow-print chaise lounge with his back to me, like I'm his psychiatrist. I figure he will be more honest with his answers if he can't see me. I had no plans to outsource this interview and miss out on red wine or a bit of Cudlee Creek (winky face)!

'I don't think your illness puts pressure on the relationship,' Matt says. 'It changes some of the dynamics, like placing some limitations on what we do and how we do it so it doesn't wipe you out, like outings and holidays. It makes us plan things differently, and it makes me think more selflessly.

'I guess the hardest thing is watching the pain you're in and not being able to do anything about it. And from that, I have to think ahead to plan around that pain and try to make things less of a burden for you, if I can. It's never going to completely make things perfect for you. And sometimes you know the pain is going to strike, but sometimes it can come without warning, and I can see how that frustrates you. It's not nice, because you'd like a body that works, and you're a very active, energetic person, and you like to be able to focus those energies.'

He's right. I get really frustrated if I can't do things. And as I get older, I can do even less. But he's very patient and we've been through a lot together.

'You do push through, but it might mean that if we've planned a lovely weekend away or something, your enjoyment of that might be curtailed by an onset of pain. And speaking more broadly too, there's been the wider struggle that it's brought to our lives: the ectopic pregnancies and the miscarriages, which have obviously been horrible things for us to go through; to watch you go through, but also to experience as a couple,' he says.

We don't know if the miscarriages were caused by the endo or adeno, because there's not enough research and knowledge in that area just now. But I was informed that I have Antiphospholipid antibodies, which are associated with recurrent miscarriage before ten weeks. And there is plenty of research to show that women who have endometriosis have an increased risk of ectopic pregnancy. An ectopic pregnancy is when a fertilised egg implants itself outside the womb. About one or two in one hundred pregnancies in Australia are ectopic, and endo patients are at a higher risk.

'That's the hardest thing,' Matt says. 'Wondering if, had you been diagnosed earlier, if things could have been quite different for you and for us. I know it's hard for you to accept it, because of course it is. It's hard for us as a couple as well.

'When you finally got a diagnosis, that was a relief, because we knew what it was, and it explained a lot. I know for you, you've been able to look back at things, and it's made a lot of sense. So obviously in that period where we didn't know what it was there was a lot of frustration.'

But to get from that point to where we are now has been a journey of positive discovery coupled with endless frustration. Due to pregnancy losses (and subsequent bodily carnage), my condition has become worse, which has meant the goalposts shift quite often.

'It's not that I don't know how to help you; there are things that I know I can do to help you and I'm doing those and it is helping you. But when you're struck down with pain or unable to do what you want to do, there's nothing I can do to stop that, and that's frustrating. To see the person that you love most in the world debilitated and not being able to do anything about that . . .' Matt sighs.

'In some ways that must be a lonely thing for you to go through. But if all I can do is show you I'm here with you in that, and loving you through everything, then hopefully it helps. But you refuse to back down and you will never go to the emergency room, because you say you don't want to waste their time, so I feel very helpless. It's horrible to watch someone you love in pain.'

He's right. I don't like going to hospital, particularly emergency, because of years of seeking help and being dismissed. In fact, I didn't even go to hospital with most of my pregnancy losses unless I was given direct instructions by the doctor, because I am so scarred from a lifetime of being sent home without any help. I have built up an incredible pain tolerance, which is probably quite unhealthy, physically and mentally. If you're a psychologist and you're reading this, clear your schedule and hit me up. I've got issues.

Pain is an everyday occurrence for Matt and me. Mostly, I just try to push through it, even if means I'll crash and burn later. I just don't want to miss out on anything. I want to live as much as I can and I hate being a burden.

'It's a strange thing where it's so much a part of our lives now,' Matt agrees. 'Like, you would be in the kind of pain that would probably send most people to hospital, but you take some anti-inflammatories or you lie down for a bit, and then you push through and get on with it. I think for both of us, we perhaps accept the pain too much. But you have to, otherwise you just stop living your life. But to the outside world it could make that seem a little uncaring, the way that we deal with it sometimes.'

We also joke a lot about endo and really poke fun at it. When we wrote our two comedy cabaret shows, *Endo The Road* and then *Endo Days,* the best part was writing songs together in the loungeroom about periods, pain, butt drugs, period leaks and dismissive doctors. We had so much fun putting the show together and performing it for the endo community – and letting them laugh at us and, in turn, themselves.

In our everyday life, we make very rude and inappropriate jokes about my condition which we've enjoyed sharing on stage. (Within reason. Some jokes aren't for public consumption, you know?) But as well as laughing, joking and performing in all-singing, all-dancing endo extravaganzas, sometimes we get really pissed off about this illness. And other times, we do what we can to raise awareness and help other people with it.

'It's terrible. You've got this condition, and it's not curable, but it's not the end of life as you know it. There are things that can be done to manage it, and it does come in cycles. So it's important to make the most of the good times, the times that you're free from it, because there will be days when things aren't great, both physically and emotionally,' Matt says. 'I mean, I could say endo brought us closer together, but I think we were already pretty close. If you didn't have it, it would probably change maybe some of the things we'd do together, like we could go run marathons together, but I don't know if we would ever do that, so . . .'

Yeah, nah, we definitely wouldn't.

'I feel that you are the bravest person I know, because you don't let this define you; you don't let this beat you,' Matt says. 'I'm going to continue to love you and support you every day through this. It's not going to go away, but I'm proud of us as a couple and what we've built as a relationship, and as a family.

'I guess what I want for you is not to be tied down by this. I want you to be free, because you're happiest when you're free, and I know that there are always going to be good days and bad days. But the good days outnumber the bad because I love you so much.'

10
Single with Endo

sex, love and dating with chronic pain

I was already married to Matt when I was diagnosed with endo-metriosis, so my experiences as a single person were affected by pain with no name. In my twenties, I dated a lot. But was not really a one-night stand gal, because I needed to get to know the person well enough to be with them and be relaxed enough to be intimate.

I remember never wanting to rush into sex – but not for moral reasons, because I believe you should have sex if and when you're ready and want to (consensually and within the legal age limit). I guess it was the pain factor. If I was tense it would hurt, so I didn't risk it. I am very outgoing and I love hanging out with people of all genders, so I was often accused of being a 'slut' (such a silly word), which is funny, because I wasn't sleeping around, due to pelvic pain. I definitely would have if I could have!

From speed dating to online dating, as well as hooking up in clubs, dating workmates, set-ups, rebounds and having a thing for musicians, I had a lot of relationships. And with all of them I had to decide whether or not I should disclose my weird fainting and stomach pains. If they stuck around long enough, they usually encouraged me to go to a doctor which made them a co-star in the next episode of *Anything but the uterus – a journey of misdiagnosis*.

Single days with endo were easier in that I didn't have three children to run around after and I could lie on the couch watching things on telly that are not animated films I have watched 30,000 times (I'm looking at you, *Frozen* and *Frozen II*). But it was also hard, because there was no one to help me if I collapsed or fainted with pain. Also, I am an extrovert, so I need to be around people – which meant I had to make more of an effort to go out more than I do when I'm in a relationship.

My tantra tantrum

In 2010, I was single and hanging out a lot with my friend Jake, who was seeing a guy in an open relationship. We were gossiping about it over dinner one night and he showed me a photo of the guy's partner. I noticed he had the same name and sparkly blue eyes as a boy I had a huge crush on in Grade One and who I always fantasised I would meet again, and fall in love, get married and live happily ever after in a tropical island paradise.

It couldn't have been him though, because we were in Adelaide and I had met that sparkly-eyed boy in Papua New Guinea. What were the odds of it being him? For laughs, Jake sent him a message to ask if he went to school in PNG. He did! What are the odds! After a few more probing questions we discovered it was that very boy I had been dreaming of all those years!

We agreed to catch up for a coffee because the coincidence was far too great to ignore. I knew he was in a long-term relationship with a man, so I figured my romantic tropical island dreams were dashed. He wouldn't be interested in me but that was okay, because we had plenty of catching up to do and I was excited to see him. We had coffee, chatted about where our lives had taken us over the past twenty-five years or so, and he told me he was bisexual (hooray!) a musician (my weakness) and an artist (swoon). He also mentioned he was a tantric sex master (oh my god). My tropical island, blue-eyed dream boy was even better than I ever could have imagined – and I'd imagined he would be pretty damned good. He asked to see me again (yes!).

161

We agreed to meet in a week from then. I spent the entire time bursting with excitement: choosing the right dress, shoes and perfume, dreaming about the amazing tantric sex I would be having. I imagined we'd be listening to sitar on vinyl, and burning incense as we drank spicy tea, talking about our feelings and having outer-body experiences. He arrived at my place looking and smelling divine and, well, I did not think this through, because oh my lord, tantric sex goes FOREVER. Like, hours and hours and hours. Don't get me wrong, I love sex, but I am very tired and impatient and I simply do not have the time or pelvic tolerance for tantra. So, that was the end of my tropical island love affair.

Single parenting with endo: Gem's story

Gem is a single mum who has taken time off from dating because she wants to focus on raising her daughter. But she happily shared her thoughts on being on the scene when you have endo – and whether she discloses it to people she's seeing.

'Normally dating for me is just slutting around, so I don't tell people unless I absolutely have to. I mainly try and just schedule dates around my cycle,' she says. 'If someone gets close to me, I disclose it pretty quickly because the chances of me bleeding everywhere or having pain during sex is pretty high, so I like to have my partners prepared. But I feel like being single is almost easier with my endo and adenomyosis because it was so rough on my relationships.

'Two weeks of the month I was in severe pain, bleeding, emotional and depressed. Being sick as a parent sucks, but being in so much pain it's hard to lift your kid or engage and play with them is heartbreaking. Brain fog and sleeplessness haven't helped my parenting and the huge mum guilt I suffer with.'

The mum guilt is real, but we'll get to that. Right now we're talking about single life.

More single stories: Sarah and Jamila

Sarah S is a GP living with endometriosis who was diagnosed aged thirty-seven. 'I'm single, but probably more because of my job,' she says. 'It took a lot of time and effort to do my training, and then to do my on-the-job training, and then my specialty qualifications. And I'm fairly introverted anyway. So, when it comes to the people I come across in the day, the majority of them are my patients and that's just not appropriate,' she laughs. 'But at the same time, I think there's some concern around any new relationships, and how this illness will affect intimacy. That's obviously a big concern for a lot of us with it. But I'd say it's more anticipated experience rather than lived experience.

'Where other people look forward to that part of a new relationship, I'd imagine I'm not alone in worrying about it, because of having chronic pain issues. And people with pain sometimes haven't been told about the contribution of muscle spasm in the pelvic floor, because often they generally have very good symptom control. A lot of the issues that they have with intimacy actually can be solved with work on pelvic floor rather than anything hugely invasive, but, it's just not really well known.'

Hear! hear!

Jamila has been dating again after a difficult break-up where their partner and carer broke up with them three days before Christmas.

'I had known for a few months that something was not fully okay with my partner, who I'd been with for almost four years, and with whom I thought I was going to spend the rest of my life,' Jamila says.

'They were like my in-house carer and by the end of our relationship, there was imbalance between them being my carer and them being my partner and lover, which I think is really tricky when someone is disabled and someone is non-disabled in a relationship.'

Jamila is an ambulant endo patient who required a high level of care from their partner, which they had warned them about when the couple first got together.

'I would often have to say, *Can you bring my heat pack? Can you carry me to my bedroom because I can't walk that far today? Can you not go to work today because my flare is so bad, I can't be on my own?* And they would just look so pained and frustrated. They looked trapped. In the first year of our relationship when I found out I had endo, I told them this would be the rest of my life and it could get really debilitating. I gave them an out and said, *If you want to fuck off now, that's fine.* And they didn't,' Jamila says.

'I was so worried that at some point it would be too much for them, and I think it was a factor in them breaking up with me, but I don't know how much they want to admit that to themselves, because that's not a nice thing to admit. But it feels so unfair that they get to walk away when endo was such a huge part of both of our lives,' Jamila says.

Jamila says while they are giving dating a red-hot go, it's scary because of the stigma attached to living with disability and chronic illness.

'I've never been single and had to worry about disclosing my endo because I was in a relationship when I was diagnosed. Now, I'm like, *Oh, this is going to make casual sex so much more complicated.* And I use a wheelchair because of my endo now, so do I include that in my Tinder profile? Do I have a picture of me in my wheelchair? Is that going to weed out the people who can't handle it?'

It's a good question. What if Jamila didn't disclose the wheelchair in a dating profile?

'Am I going to catfish them if I don't? And is it any of their business? And am I just going to open myself up to more rejection because I have to sit down a lot? And will they just fail to appreciate how fucking excellent I am? Because I'm a fucking catch!' Jamila enthuses.

'But I don't want to have to deal with ableism. I want to have a nice drink with someone and not have to worry about whether I have to educate them or if they're going to say offensive shit to me.'

Accountable to no one: a benefit of being single with endo

Facing ableism would make dating so hard. I know when I couldn't explain why I needed to take time out to rest because my body was exhausted, that was a dealbreaker for some people. I am such a party gal the rest of the time, and they didn't like it if I needed to go underground for a while – which meant I was sometimes ghosted by people I was seeing. Even if I could have told them I was living with endo, my suspicion is they would have bailed anyway because it was too hard.

But living alone and being single with chronic pain was great for me in that I wasn't accountable to anyone. I could crash and burn when I needed to and comfort telly was always my choice, which made recovering from a flare much easier to cope with. And because I only had to clean up after and take care of myself, my pain wasn't as bad as it is now. But I remember times when I was in too much pain to get a heat pack, dinner or shopping, or I'd faint and hurt myself with no one there to help me (or at least laugh about my clumsy fall). And, while I didn't have a name for my endo, if ever I told a potential suitor I had anxiety and depression so bad it would make me pass out, they usually backed away slowly and made their exit. But that's okay, because they weren't worth the effort anyway.

Being single and coping with pain isn't easy, but there are some things you can do to take the load off (see below for tips). Whether you're in casual relationships, single and looking for a partner, or committed to independence, what you disclose and how much you share about your illness is up to you – and you shouldn't feel any pressure to give more or less of yourself than you want to. Just promise me you won't compromise your safety or comfort because you're considering someone else's feelings. Now go out there and get slutting! Or not. That's okay too. Just stay safe and look after yourself. You're the most important factor.

6 tips for coping with endo pain while single

1. Have an endo first-aid kit with medications, heat packs, tens machines and all of your endo accessories, in a spot you can reach in emergencies. Keep a fresh bottle of water in there for swallowing painkillers and don't forget you must always replenish if you borrow from the kit. It's for emergencies.

2. Keep some ready meals in the freezer, or freeze some fresh meals you can microwave if you're feeling rubbish.

3. Keep emergency numbers by the phone and identify someone in your life you can call or contact if you're in a bad way and need help.

4. Keep reminding yourself that if someone can't handle your illness, they will be intolerant of other things that are important to you, so set them free.

5. Have a brief explanation ready for someone you meet if you are comfortable disclosing your illness to them. It could be something like, *I have a condition called endometriosis which causes chronic pain. I have good days and bad days. Today is a <insert good/bad here> day. If you have any questions, I'd be really happy to tell you more. Otherwise, check out EndoZone, QENDO or Endometriosis Australia websites.*

6. Chat with a pelvic floor physio about how they can help you with any concerns you have about sex and intimacy. They can help you with relaxing the muscles in your pelvis and show you how to use dilators and OhNuts to make penetrative sex easier.

11

Parenting and Family Relationships with Endo

Many challenging things have happened while I've been writing this book. COVID-19 sent the world into lockdown and millions of people have lost their lives and livelihoods. I had my eleventh pregnancy loss, my third endo surgery, my beloved cat of eleven years died of aggressive bone cancer, and our family fostered a little boy.

After trying to have a baby for eight years, Matt and I made a decision to stop. We were exhausted. I was exhausted. We chose to focus on running our business and start the process of becoming carers together. Before I met Matt, I was approved to become a foster parent, but the process took about eighteen months. By the time I received my approval, Matt and I were in a relationship and I had taken on the role of co-parenting his two children, who were very young at the time. I decided to shelve the idea of foster care and come back to it later. I needed to focus on building a relationship with Niamh and Keeley.

It was wonderful welcoming the girls into my family, where they found two more cousins in my sister Kathryn's two boys Kane and Jake, a grandma and grandpa in my mum Lorraine and her partner David, as and a pop in my dad Phillip, who the girls have always called Phillip Pillip. On Matt's side, I was lucky to gain another sister in Sarah, the best mother-in-law anyone could ever ask for in Mary, and a swag of beautiful cousins, aunties, uncles and adorable babies of cousins.

'Their only desire was for me to be okay': my daughters' story

My stepdaughters have given me so much to be thankful for. They are loving, hilarious, smart, strong, talented, stubborn and compassionate people. When Matt and I started hanging out together, Niamh told him he should marry me, so he did. I loved the girls from the minute I met them and I am so lucky to be in their lives. They've watched Matt and me go through a lot – and we have gone through plenty together as a family. When they were younger, they were excited for me to give them a brother or sister to play with. But as the years went on and after all the losses, their only desire was for me to be okay.

'I wish you didn't have to go through all this pain,' Niamh (fourteen) says. 'I wish doctors had listened more, rather than being so quick to say it's in your head. I think the pain you go through scares us all sometimes and I really wish there was a cure so you would be better.

'It is challenging to see someone you love go through immense pain and loss, but also it has brought us closer together as a family and because we've talked about it, I know a lot more about endo and chronic illness, so I can help people who have it.'

Niamh is a clever, resilient, ambitious young person with compassion that knows no bounds. She hates injustice, is fiercely loyal and is the nicest person I have ever known. If I was half the person Niamh is, I would be very fortunate indeed.

Keeley is creative, hilarious, kind, caring, adventurous and thoughtful. She loves animals, music and being with the people she adores. Keeley is such a warm and affectionate kid, whose friendship and love I feel so privileged to receive.

When I interviewed both girls, they spoke candidly – particularly Keeley, who had just woken up and was extremely honest in her sleep state.

'I mean, having a mum with endometriosis is not that different to having a mum who doesn't have endometriosis,' Keeley (eleven) says. 'It doesn't stop you from doing things. You do them anyway. You probably shouldn't do that. It's not that good for you. You probably shouldn't push yourself as much, but that's kind of your thing.'

Yeah, it is kind of my thing.

At this point, I need to let you know that both girls call their dad 'Doy'. (When she was little, Keeley used to call Matt 'Daddoy', which then shortened to Doy and we've all called him Doy ever since.)

'I don't remember many of your hospital visits,' Keeley muses, 'except for sharing your hospital food with you and watching *The Lorax* on the TV in your hospital bed. I also remember you coming home from hospital and doing things when you should have been resting and Doy telling you to rest, but you never do.'

Kids, eh? So honest!

I was really worried the girls would see me in pain and that would cause them to worry about getting their periods, thinking everyone goes through what I do. We talked about it a lot and I made sure they were completely prepared when the time came. We read books, went through the clinical and anecdotal stuff about periods, and normalised the whole function of menstruating. I asked them recently if they had been scared of menstruation. Their answers genuinely surprised me.

'No, I wasn't scared at all to get my period, because we talked about it so much and we were so open about period stuff,' Niamh says.

'Nope. I wasn't scared. You talked to us a lot about it. Like, a *lot*,' Keeley laughs. 'And sometimes you have bad pain but when you do, you sit on the couch, so I get to sit on the couch with you and we can hang out and watch movies together.'

Silver lining, I guess. Keeley always sees the bright side of things. When she was about six and we were in the car, I was getting grumpy about the number of red lights we were getting and she said, 'We have to wait here, but it means that we get to spend more time together!' That outlook has helped me through many dark days.

Both of my stepdaughters have used our experiences and turned them into positives. Niamh is a real freedom fighter and she sees my condition as a chance to raise awareness and change the world.

'If any of my friends had bad pain like you, I would tell them to go to the doctor, but if the doctor ignores them, I would tell them what I know about endo and then tell them to go and see another doctor. Because if you think something is wrong with your body, then it's likely that there is something wrong. It's your body and you know when something's wrong with you so you shouldn't accept it if anyone tries to tell you that you aren't feeling what you're feeling,' she says.

I am thrilled that this is what she's taken from all our talking, singing, writing of education programs and conversation about period pain and endometriosis. I am so proud she's lived our experiences and is using the information to make the world a better place. She's such a fantastic kid.

And while our whole family is busily making lemonade from all the lemons, there are some things that stand out and have affected them, which makes me sad. There are challenges we've gone through that have changed us.

'Normally you are okay and you just tell us when you aren't feeling well, but one time we were in the kitchen and Doy was downstairs. Niamh was doing her homework. You were cooking and I was helping you, but you were having a bad pain day and you fainted and hit your head on the counter and then you fell down. I had to yell out for Doy and I was scared. I didn't think you were okay,' Keeley says.

I remember that day very well and I cannot get her little voice out of my head, panicked and shouting, 'Daddoy! Daddoy!' Matt came running. I tried to get up to pretend everything was okay so I wouldn't scare her, but I fell back down again and hit the back of my head on the floor. Keeley grabbed the little stool she used to stand on to help me in the kitchen and she put it under my head. She put some tea towels over me to keep me warm. That was about two years after my diagnosis. It was at that point I realised if I didn't get this pain under control, I was going to have a bad accident or do some real damage.

Chatting with both girls about everything from health to consent, friendships to goals and ambitions, has been so enlightening for me. In the house I grew up in, we didn't really talk about these things. It's been such a pleasure to be able to have open, honest and supportive conversations about stuff in their lives and ours. I always wanted a close and loving household filled with children. It never occurred to me I might not be able to have children. I've been so lucky to have Niamh and Keeley and I have never thought of them as anything other than my children. I love them more than I ever imagined it was possible and I am so proud of who they are.

Not a wicked stepmother

Being a stepmother isn't easy. There's a giant stigma attached to it. The Wicked Stepmother trope follows us around. At the girls' Catholic primary school, I was always excluded from the mum catch-ups, and the drop-off and pick-up gossip circles. I didn't care so much about that, because I met some great mums who were also outcasts and they were far more fun. Also, the girls' mum would always pass on invitations to school events that were for mums only, which was lovely and appreciated. But sometimes my exclusion really hurt the kids, which is unacceptable.

Niamh had the same teacher for three years in a row. For some reason, this teacher absolutely refused to acknowledge me as Niamh's parent, despite me dropping the girls off and picking them up every week for seven years – not to mention going to assemblies, gatherings, parent-teacher interviews, concerts and all the rest. Each year, the students made presents for Mother's Day and each year, Niamh asked to make two because she said she has two mums. Each year, her teacher said no.

But it wasn't just the teachers. One year Keeley had a birthday party and we invited all her friends for go-karting, laser skirmish and arcade games, then back to our place for a sleepover. Three out of the five girls weren't allowed to sleep over. One girl told Keeley (who told me), 'Mum said I can't stay because it's not at your real mum's house and she doesn't know your other mum.' (Remember, I did school pick up and drop off, concerts, assemblies and all the rest. I was at the school every single week.) I was hurt. Keeley was hurt. But we focused on the positives and made it the greatest party of all time.

When the anti-sleepover mums arrived at the party (together, of course), one of them took one look at me and said, 'Oh, I know you! I've seen you at school!' and I nervously chuckled and said, 'Yes, I've been around quite a long time now.' Another anti-sleepover mum agreed and laughed, 'We probably could have let them sleep over and had a night off!' Yeah, they probably could have. I hope they learned a lesson in judging people who aren't in traditional, nuclear family settings, though I doubt it. Still, it was a great party, we had a blast and Keeley still talks about it. Sucked in, anti-sleepover mums. You missed out.

Another time, the receptionist at the kids' school was on the phone asking the sports coordinator a question about touch football on my behalf. I was trying to find out where the game was being held so I could go and watch Niamh play – you know, like parents do. The sports coordinator on the other end of the line must have asked for whom she was asking and the receptionist looked me up and down and hissed down the phone, 'It's Niamh's, um, Niamh's, um . . . yeah.' When we left the room with the touch footy information, and me with a very red face, Niamh said, 'You're not my "Um Yeah", you're my Hell Yeah!'. Which was actually one of the best things anyone has ever said to me.

I know there are some Wicked Stepmothers out there. I realise break-ups are hard, and people want to choose sides. But two happy households are better than one unhappy household. Niamh and Keeley have two mums they can look to for guidance and advice, and three parents who absolutely love them to bits. If you want to choose sides, choose the kids' side. Champion their happiness.

I've never felt like the girls aren't my kids, even before I discovered I wasn't able to birth my own. As a teacher, I cared a lot for every single student I worked with. And when Matt and I started dating, I would bring craft, dress-ups and games for the girls every time they were around. We always hung out together as a family and when they come to our place, it's my favourite time of the week. When I married Matt, I married into their lives, so we always celebrate our wedding anniversary as a family. I hope that will never change.

What's a 'real' mum?

Matt and I made the decision to foster a child after we cancelled our IVF treatment. We asked for Niamh and Keeley's blessing first. If they didn't want it, we wouldn't have pursued it. But they were thrilled to have an opportunity to open their home to a child in need of the love and care we have to offer.

Now we are a family of five and life is beautifully hectic, hard, rewarding, silly . . . and did I mention hectic?

We had just finished up a ten-show run at Adelaide Fringe when we were told (after eighteen months of training, screening, security checks and home safety clearances) that a little boy would be coming to live with us. A two-year-old who will be with us long-term. We knew very little about this tiny guy and had to learn very quickly what he likes, doesn't like, what he eats, when he sleeps, and most importantly, what he needs to feel safe and loved.

This baby has absolutely captured our hearts. We couldn't love him any harder if we tried. He has the best big sisters in the whole world and I am pouring everything I have into helping him catch up on his growth, development and sense of security.

Every morning when we hear his tiny footsteps running into our room to give us a big squeeze, through to every night when we kiss his beautiful little face goodnight, I feel so lucky he has come to us.

He fills our house with such joy and though he has no idea, he is mending my very, very broken heart. I know I'm not his 'real mum'. But what is a real mum? I am a real mum to my girls and to my boy – and their 'real mums' are mums to them as well. Everyone is mumming as well as they are able to. We all do it differently and most of us are just doing our best.

Does being a mum mean you pushed a baby out your vagina? What about caesareans then? Does being a mum mean your kids call you 'mum'? Because my girls call me Yib, Yibby, Siba, Yobby, Sibsib and Hell Yeah and they call their father Doy or Monkey Man (because when he wears headphones to record music, he apparently looks like a monkey). Does being a mum mean you're with your kids all the time? Or does it mean you love them to bits when you see them at your access visit, or your allocated days, or when they come to visit from out of town? Being a mum is less about DNA and so much more about love. It's about showing up, stepping up and loving the shit out of whoever you are privileged to care for.

For stepmums, foster mums, carers and anyone else taking on a mother role to children, being excluded from the Real Mum™ Club is hard. But it's even worse when you've tried your hardest to have babies. I work hard to keep a positive and sunny disposition in the face of adversity, but it hurts when people discount my role in my three kids' lives. And the kids see it, too. They hear people saying I'm not their real mum, and it invalidates their feelings and their family.

'You are the best stepmum in the world, because you love and care for us like we're your children, and we are,' Keeley says. 'You are so kind to [Little Guy], Niamh and me.'

I asked one of the mothers who let her daughter sleep over at Keeley's birthday party why she took a chance on a stepmum when the others didn't. 'I look at the kids,' she said. 'They're happy, safe, healthy. Look at the kids and you see who the parents are.'

Despite the challenges we've faced as a family, we are solid and we will always communicate to make sure all our children feel valued and respected.

When the little guy came to live with us, I'd had another endo surgery not long beforehand. The physical demands of a toddler can be brutal when you're living with chronic pain. But it has been a case of mind over matter. I push through the pain and all the other mantras to get through the day, put him to bed and then collapse under the weight of my illness until I get up and do it again tomorrow. He keeps me moving, he keeps me laughing and he reminds me how much love I have to give.

Parenting with endo

Parenting is hard. Parenting with endo is a whole other level of hard. Parenting with endo when your children also have endo would also be heartbreaking.

Endometriosis is thought to have a genetic predisposition, and there are studies examining familial patterns and endometriosis. But as always, this is an underfunded and under-researched area of health, so there is still a lot to learn and discover about this. Anecdotally, though, many of the people I speak with say their mothers, sisters, aunties and grandmothers are diagnosed with endo or have lived with symptoms.

As an administrator of the South Australian endo support group on Facebook, I often see mothers desperately seeking answers, support and treatment for their children. They don't want them to go through what they went through.

Closer to home, my best mate Amy is a parent of three, including a toddler. She says parenting with endo is a whole body and mind experience.

'It's full-body exhaustion. It's needing extra rest all the time and having to cancel plans. It's pushing through the pain and not being able to take time off, ever,' she says.

Two of Amy's children are assigned female at birth, but the eldest (fifteen) identifies as male and the youngest (thirteen) as non-binary. Both have watched their mum go through her pain episodes and hormone fluctuations. Amy feared they may end up the same way. Endometriosis is strongly influenced by genetic factors, so people who menstruate who have a family history of endo are more likely to develop it. Some studies say fifty per cent of the risk factors for endo are genetic.

'I was always concerned that they would have it and I would wish so hard that they wouldn't,' she says. 'It was so hard knowing how much endo pain I had to endure, as well as not knowing if I could cope with watching my babies experience the same traumatic pain episodes that I had. They would also ask me, *Will my period hurt me like it hurts you?* And I couldn't promise that it wouldn't.'

Vanessa's daughter Annabel (fourteen) hasn't shown any signs of endo as yet, but they are both prepared if that day should come. You met Vanessa back in Chapter Seven. She's the dentist who started the South Australian endo support group.

'My daughter knows everything about periods and endometriosis because it's all around her. So now she's got the tools. She's informed. If she has period pains and maybe they're not normal, she'll know to speak up,' she says.

Vanessa says her daughter's education and mental toolkit are the silver linings of her own endometriosis. It means she is more compassionate and has sympathy for other people with pain.

Supporting your endo kid

Endometriosis Australia's Donna Ciccia has helped countless patients, partners and parents with advice and guidance. She says offering a healthy balance of independence and support is the best way to help a chronically ill person.

'If you're a supporter, you need to just be there. Just listen. You're not there to fix it. You're not there to make things happen or take on all of their appointments. You're there to learn and to listen.

'For parents who have kids with endo, you have to empower them, as opposed to do it for them. You want them to be able to be independent enough to make good decisions and to be empowered. I really encourage people to not be the passenger. Don't let someone else take control, because you won't ever get better. You need to be engaged and part of the journey, not just along for the journey.'

Lesley and Syl's story: closer and more empowered

EndoActive mother and daughter Lesley and Syl became closer and more empowered through their discovery of Syl's condition. They are determined, driven and resourceful. And Lesley has learned how to help her daughter live with this illness while creating an online community for patients.

'I never went to the doctor about period pain because Mum said periods were meant to be painful,' Syl says. 'We never got told any differently at school. I didn't really have any reason to think that there was anything worthwhile going to the doctor about, I just hated getting my period because it was sore. But I obviously started to get a lot sicker and I didn't know anything about immune systems and pelvic pain and fatigue, and how to manage any type of symptoms through diet or anything.

'Eventually what led to the diagnosis was my UTIs were getting more and more chronic (this is chronic cystitis) and then I said something, in jest, to Mum about light bladder leakage when I was twenty-one. And she was like, *Yeah, that's not normal*. And so that's why we went to go see a uro-gynaecologist who wound up diagnosing me with endo. That was the first time anyone had really asked me about my history with period pain in a medical appointment.'

'Totally shocked me,' Syl's mother Lesley says. 'I'd heard of old ladies or people who've had several children getting light bladder leakage, but not young girls. I never heard of endo either, but if she had a really bad pain, I would drive her to school or pick her up. I remember occasionally we'd go to the movies with a hot water bottle.'

Lesley says that if she'd known 'even a third' of the information she and Syl provide in the educational videos on EndoActive's website, it would have made a huge difference. 'We'd have been so much better prepared. Everything for us was the first time.'

The difficult thing is that we don't have enough information available for people with endo. There's a fear of giving people misinformation because stuff that's available is often anecdotal or isn't supported by research – because the research doesn't exist, or it's really scientific and not accessible for endo patients.

And while none of us have enough answers, Syl and Lesley have worked hard together to improve the lives of others, and Lesley has been a huge support to Syl. For parents who are caring for a child with endo or suspected endo, Syl recommends looking at it holistically.

'Look beyond the obvious symptoms of endo. Look at all the symptoms and different ailments, not as isolated events. Ask yourself, is my child tired? Getting migraines? Getting infections all the time? Or things that are hard to get rid of? Compromised immune system? Digestion issues? All those things, beyond just period flow and period pain, can all be an indication that your child's not well. And it might not be with endo: it might be some type of autoimmune deficiency or disorder,' Syl says.

'And obviously, believe their pain and be their health advocate, because a lot of the time when you're sick with endo or with chronic illness, the brain fog is so severe. And as a kid, you don't know how to navigate a healthcare system anyway. So, you really need an adult.'

6 tips for supporting a family member with endo:

1. Believe them.
2. Accompany them to appointments and take notes for them.
3. Make accommodations and allowances for them to be comfortable at events.
4. Check in with them to see if they need anything.
5. Educate yourself about endo.

6. Keep up to date with the latest, which means reading articles yourself, not tagging an endo patient in the comments section of a post on social media because you saw the word 'endo' in it. I've been tagged in articles I've actually authored because a well-meaning person has thought *Ooh, endo! Libby would be interested in this!* without actually reading it first.

We're not making this up!

In a perfect world, people would just believe us, wouldn't they? At the end of one of my shows, a group of women were standing in a circle, crying. That's not generally the response I want after a comedy show, so I headed over to chat with them. I wanted to see which song or joke I should cut to avoid further upset.

But what I found was a circle of women who had come to support their young relative and had only just realised they had dismissed her for the entirety of her illness thus far. 'We didn't believe her,' one woman said, sobbing. The others nodded, clutching tissues, holding each other's hands. 'But after hearing your story and the stories of the other women in the room, we are so, so sorry.' They turned to her, 'We are so, so sorry.' Then we were all crying.

Another night, a woman who was sitting with her daughter put up her hand and asked to share. It is that kind of show, so it was fine. She said she felt terrible because she didn't believe her daughter when she first complained about her pain. She cried. I didn't know what else to say, so I said, 'But you're here now.' And then – again – we were all crying.

It's a huge relief to us when people finally validate our feelings, pain and illness. But why does it take so long? Why is it so hard to believe people in pain? Once you get past assumptions that you are attention-seeking, task-avoiding, anxious, or drug-seeking, how can you convince a person you are genuinely ill if they can't see your illness? People don't question someone wearing a cast on their arm or a moon boot.

From friendships to family, endo can put the pressure on. But if you don't feel supported, or if someone doesn't believe your pain, you can set some boundaries to keep yourself safe.

5 tips for helping your friends and family to help with your endo:

1. Give them some links to some websites, like EndoZone, Endometriosis Australia, QENDO, Jean Hailes, EndoActive or PPFA. Ask them to speak to you about it when they've had a look, so you can discuss any questions they might have.

2. Keep them in the loop when you aren't feeling well. Communication is key. If you don't tell them what's happening, they will assume. And that's not going to be helpful.

3. Tell them what you need, but also tell them what you don't need. For example, I don't respond to 'tough love'. If I'm feeling unwell and having a doona day, I will respond very badly to someone saying, *come on, get up, you'll feel better if you get moving.* I know what I need and I'll do it, thank you very much. I don't always make the best choices for myself, but pausing under a quilt for a day never hurt anyone!

4. Be patient with them. They can't possibly understand what you're going through if they aren't dealing with it themselves.

5. Set your boundaries and only do things that are within your capability and capacity. If you can't go to Aunty Pam's birthday party because you are having a pain flare-up, Aunty Pam will get over it. It's better than going along, being miserable and not explaining why, so Aunty Pam assumes it's because you hate the cheesecake she made.

12
Loss and Debacle

Trigger warning: *pregnancy loss*

I touched on it earlier, but to refresh: my endo was discovered after an ectopic pregnancy. This was the first of eleven pregnancy losses I have suffered over seven years. I don't normally like to use the word 'suffered' because I prefer the word 'survived' or 'lived with', so as to empower others and myself. But in this case, I am going to allow myself the words and the space to call it what it is: suffering a loss.

I also don't like the word 'miscarriage'. To me, it sounds like I've done something wrong. When there has been a failure of a court or judicial system, then that's a miscarriage of justice. While writing this, when I right-click > synonym on the word 'miscarriage', I can select from the following: failure, lapse, breakdown, insufficiency, mistake, blunder, debacle.

Debacle! Well, pregnancy loss can certainly be disastrous, but the word 'miscarriage' makes it sound like the carrier of the pregnancy has made a mistake; that the blame lies with them. I may seem to be reading too much into it. But strap yourself in, because I'm going even deeper.

Before I do though, if pregnancy loss is triggering for you, please skip to the next chapter. I'm going to share some stories that may be distressing for you and it's important to keep yourself safe. But you are not alone and I understand what you are feeling. So, draw yourself a bath and make yourself a cup of tea (or a wine-flavoured beverage) and come back when I'm talking more about butts and poo and tantric sex and stuff.

Pregnancy loss, shame and being alone with the pain

Anyone who has suffered a pregnancy loss will understand the blame and shame that is attached to it. When you fall pregnant, there is a rule that you wait until the first trimester is over before you tell people about it, in case you miscarry. This has always confused me. Possibly because I am a person who absolutely, under no circumstances, can keep a secret. But also because that means you go through the first part of your pregnancy alone (well, presumably your partner or co-parent would know). And then, should you lose your pregnancy, you also go through that loss alone.

Pregnancy loss makes people uncomfortable. I know that far too well. I have lost dozens of friends because my inability to sustain a pregnancy in my body makes them feel bad, especially when they are having babies or announcing pregnancies. (Sometimes they come to me when they have a pregnancy loss, but then get pregnant again and carry to full term. And then feel guilty that I haven't had that, so they just stop communicating with me and the friendship is over). I get it; really, I do. They didn't want to make me feel bad, so they backed off. But when they do that, I feel bad that they felt uncomfortable, and then we all feel awful – and I've lost another friend, through no fault of my own. But what can I do?

I would give anything to have been able to birth one of the eleven pregnancies my body has started. All my life I have wanted to be a mother. Even after every loss, I never gave up hope, because I so desperately wanted a family. As the years passed and my biological clock tick-tocked, I thought, *I'll give myself until I'm forty-two years old and then I'll stop.* As my forty-second birthday approached, I was filled with despair. It hadn't happened. I was exhausted. My body was tired and damaged. Matt was tired too.

Now I'm trying to give up trying to have my own baby. I have two gorgeous stepkids, a foster son and a husband who have had to watch me live through every loss. If not for my sake, for their sakes, I need to stop. I understand that now I will never birth my own child. This unimaginable grief is something I never thought I would have to endure. And yet, here we are. I don't know if I will ever get over it or find a way to accept it, but if being vocal about pregnancy loss helps other people feel less shame and less alone, I'll keep shouting about it.

The little guy we are fostering is certainly filling a hole in my heart. I tell him and my girls they are enough. And they are. But the pain in my heart from all those lost babies takes up a lot of space. I try to believe that one day I'll be healed. That one day I'll realise I've spent days, weeks, months or even years without hurting. But for now, I barely go an hour without a reminder that I can't have a baby.

My fertility journey

But it doesn't help that I am so damned good at falling pregnant. The story of my fertility journey starts at Adelaide Fringe Festival 2013 – a year prior to my endo diagnosis. I was directing a show for a local theatre company. My husband, Matt, was the lead actor, the cast were wonderful, and I was in a good place in my life. Matt and I had been living together for about a year.

We were planning to get married and have a family, to add a sibling for his two gorgeous daughters. He and his previous partner had no issues falling pregnant and I had no reason to believe my body was going to give us any trouble, so we set a date for when we'd start trying. I adjusted my private health insurance, we bought some baby stuff, we had supplies from Matt's young kids to use as hand-me-downs. We had it all worked out. We fell pregnant the first moment we tried. *That was easy!* I thought. I was pretty cocky, actually. Years later, I would often obsess about whether my cockiness brought me bad luck to the tune of seven years' recurrent miscarriage. (See what I mean about the blame and the shame?)

Because I had lived all of my menstruating life in pain and because I had no real idea what pregnancy felt like, I was not worried when I was in terrible pain and feeling rotten. *That's just being pregnant, right?* I mused, rubbing my belly, ordering more baby stuff and feeling butterflies about the prospect of welcoming a new little person into our home. But I was also passing out, having horrendous nightmares and suffering severe pain on the left side of my body, from my pelvis to my shoulder. *I just need to get through directing the show and I'll go to the doctor,* I promised myself.

But the cast was getting annoyed with how vague I was, because my brain wasn't working properly. I was not on my game. They didn't know I was pregnant, because I was following that all-important first trimester secrecy rule. I wish I had told them though, because I reckon a couple of the mums might have been able to spot the issue earlier than I did. I passed out several times and was in so much pain I could barely walk: any weight placed on my left side would send sparks of pain up and down my body.

After the show wrapped, I was at the newspaper sales job I hated, and I finally confessed to a friend that I thought something wasn't right. 'Stop being negative,' she said. 'Everything is fine, you're just worrying for nothing.' But another woman overheard our conversation and whispered, 'If you're worried, go to a doctor, now. What have you got to lose? If it's fine, it's fine. If it's not, at least you're in the right place.'

I decided to sit on it for a while, but my body had other ideas. I started to bleed; just the tiniest amount, but enough to make me call my doctor, who told me to come in immediately.

Matt came to pick me up and we spent the entire car ride trying to convince ourselves everything was fine. But the minute the doctor put his hand on my abdomen, I almost leaped off the table and I was sent directly to the hospital with a suspected ectopic pregnancy. I couldn't fight the tears. I wanted to howl, but I didn't want to upset anyone in the doctor's waiting room.

We arrived at the private hospital and the doctor had called ahead, so they were expecting me. I was grateful for the VIP treatment, but it was all happening so fast and I was rushed in for tests, scans, pokes and prods. We tried to remain positive, and so did a cheery nurse who said, *Pish posh, you'll be absolutely fine! I have a good feeling about this. I reckon baby will be right as rain!* That made us smile and we tried to convince ourselves that everything was fine. But the whispers from the medical team were deafeningly loud:

'I can't see anything in her uterus and I can't see anything in her tube.'

'Is she absolutely sure she's pregnant?'

'She says she is.'

'We tested her, she's definitely pregnant.'

I could hear the urgent whispers from the bed I lay on, with Matt by my side. My heart was racing. What was happening? All of our plans and all of my dreams were crashing down around us. We kept hearing the word 'ectopic', which I understood well, because my sister had an ectopic pregnancy. But the obstetrician kept saying, 'cornual'. We know now that a cornual ectopic is a rare form of ectopic pregnancy where the embryo implants in a cavity, or in my case, the outside corner of the uterus. But at the time, we couldn't understand what was happening and the doctors couldn't confirm with a scan, because it seemed to be very complicated. Cornual pregnancy represents only two to four per cent of tubal (ectopic) pregnancies and occurs around once in every 2500–5000 live births. At the time, though, I had no idea what they were talking about.

I had to go into surgery immediately, but my private health insurance wouldn't cover me because I had organised for my pregnancy cover to kick in when the baby was to be born. It never occurred to me that I might need it sooner. (Did I jinx it? I obsessed over that as well.) The nurse who delivered that news cried as she told me I wasn't covered and that we would have to leave the hospital, go home, pack a bag and meet the surgeon (who we know as Dr iPad) at the nearest public hospital, where we'd have to wait until an operating theatre was available.

'It'll just be a quick keyhole surgery,' Dr iPad said. 'Shouldn't take long, but it's important we get this out straight away.'

I went into surgery at 1am the Wednesday before the Easter long weekend. We were meant to be going to a concert that night. I had lunch with friends booked for the next day. I worried about how I would make sure the Easter Bunny would visit the kids, who were three and five at the time.

I woke up the next morning with a bandage across my abdomen. The nurse came in and took my blood pressure and temperature, and offered painkillers. I asked what had happened, because it didn't look like keyhole surgery to me. She went white and said, 'Oh, hasn't the doctor spoken to you? I will get him to visit you.' My immediate (and in hindsight very catastrophic) thought was I'd been given an emergency hysterectomy, because it was very clear I had been opened up in what appeared to be (with my extensive medical knowledge, thanks to shows like *A Country Practice, House* and *Grey's Anatomy*) a C-section.

Matt called from home. He hadn't been permitted to wait at the hospital with me. He eased my hysterectomy hysteria and told me the procedure had been too complicated to perform by keyhole. Dr iPad said he was too tired, so he did it via caesarean. When the doctor came to see me that morning, he showed me countless pictures of my uterus (on his iPad, of course), which was blue and swollen from decay. He laughed and called my uterus, 'a big, blue, rotting sausage'. I didn't laugh.

Fun fact: when one is hospitalised for anything related to pregnancy loss, one is housed in the maternity ward. I cannot properly describe to you what it feels like to hear newborn babies cry and families excitedly meeting their new nephew/niece/grandchild/sibling when you're lying in a hospital bed nursing a broken heart and a surgically removed pregnancy. I simply do not have words to explain what that does to a person. But, as a rule, Matt and I use dark humour to defuse difficult situations and we joked that while other people were visited with balloons that said, 'It's a boy!' or 'It's a girl!', we could have had one that said, 'It's a blue sausage!'

I was in hospital for five or maybe six days, I can't remember. I missed Easter with my stepdaughters and I didn't get to be the bunny. I didn't leave my bed much and I ran out of tears to cry. Good friends came to see me. My stepdaughters climbed into my hospital bed and watched *The Lorax* with me. They still remember it, but they didn't really understand why I was there. They always remembered it as a fun time because they got to eat the jelly that was delivered to my room, and run around in the kids' play area at the hospital. In my memory, it was a dark time of pain, sadness, loneliness, confusion and so much self-blame.

Because I had been so occupied with directing my show, and because I didn't bother to acknowledge my pain and my health, and because I had been to doctors with my pain for years only to be told there was nothing wrong with me, I had not looked after myself. I allowed a cornual ectopic pregnancy to sit on my uterus and decay for nine weeks. And because we don't talk about pregnancy in the first trimester, I couldn't ask anyone whether the pain, the passing out and the pinching feeling in my shoulder were normal.

So, I now say, sod that. Talk about it. Ask if things are normal. Ask people who've been through it. Lean on each other. Give each other comfort, advice, warnings and support.

A year after that operation – an incredibly difficult year – I was diagnosed with endometriosis (see chapter one). I asked the doctor why he didn't notice the lesions when he had me open in surgery twelve months earlier and he said he wasn't looking for it. Fair enough, I guess. He had his hands full with removing part of my big, blue sausage.

I fell pregnant a couple more times after that and lost the pregnancies early. Then, in 2015, I fell pregnant and it seemed to be sticking around. I did all the right things and got tested immediately. I chose a new doctor, who I don't have a funny name for, because it's a really unfunny story. This new doctor seemed very hopeful and confident, because my hormone levels (hCG) were doubling every day. (Which usually indicates a healthy pregnancy.) I was excited. Matt was excited. Could this be the one?

Then I started to bleed. Just the tiniest amount. But enough that I tried to visit my new doctor. It was difficult. The admin staff said I was fussing over nothing but they would try to fit me in. I told them of my recurrent miscarriage situation and they begrudgingly made room for me on the schedule. A different examination room, a different nurse, a new doctor, but the same story.

'I'm sorry, this is a non-viable pregnancy.'

I cried. We cried. The nurse cried. I felt insanely guilty. What was I doing so wrong? I felt inadequate. Everyone around me was falling pregnant and staying pregnant. Why couldn't I? I felt angry. It wasn't fair.

'It should pass through in a week or so. If it gets scary or doesn't pass through by then, give us a call,' the doctor said. And he sent us on our way.

It gets scary? I thought. *How? Why?* But I was too sad to ask. And besides, what could be scarier than a cornual ectopic?

It was close to Christmas. I was a teacher at the time, and we were just wrapping up the school year. I took a couple of days off and waited for the miscarriage to happen. It didn't. The doctor told me he'd do a 'quick curette' so I could get on with my life. I was so grateful. Two days after a very fast and pretty uneventful curette, I went back to work. I was a senior secondary teacher at a High Fee-Paying School, so my Year Eleven and Twelve students had finished for the year and I was prepping for the new year. But I was sad and feeling awful, and I didn't want to talk to anyone about my recent absence, so I chose to take myself off to work in another area of the school for some solitude.

As I climbed the concrete flight of stairs up to the library, a lovely colleague walked past, called out to me from the below quadrangle and waved. I turned to wave back and the next thing I remember is waking up at the foot of the stairs, everything aching, my trousers torn and my face bleeding. I must have only been out for a few seconds, but when I woke, a couple of year nine boys had run to my aid and were trying to rouse me, asking each other, 'Is she dead?' I told them to find someone to help me up the stairs so I could hide my embarrassment and my ripped pants. They were very kind to me.

Someone called Matt to come and pick me up. I was a mess. Both my ankles were twisted and swollen. My knee was swollen and all the skin had come off, almost down to the bone. My face escaped much damage; it was just my chin and lip that were grazed. It was then that I started to bleed – soaking a maxi-pad every half hour. I thought that was strange, because it was only a short time after my curette and I wouldn't have thought there was anything left inside me. But when I called the doctor's office, they seemed unfazed and told me it was completely normal and perhaps I had 'stirred something up when I fell over'. I asked to speak to the doctor, but they said he was busy, so I trusted their word and rested.

It was Matt's fortieth birthday and I could do nothing to celebrate. I could barely walk because my ankles and knees were still damaged and I was so dizzy all the time. Friends came over with cake and presents for him, which they had bought on my behalf. Some people are so incredibly thoughtful. As a person who finds it virtually impossible to accept help from anyone, this was overwhelming. In particular, my friend Jessie, whenever I miscarry, brings over pregnancy contraband like soft cheeses, shellfish and wine. Everyone needs a friend like Jessie.

In the days after the fall, I was violently ill and dizzy all the time but the admin staff at the doctor's office told me over the phone everything was okay and still wouldn't let me speak to the doctor. So Matt suggested I go out and do something to cheer me up. I went out to dinner and a Christmas movie with Jessie and, after vomiting in the bathroom and then passing out in my chair in the cinema, she insisted I called my doctor on his mobile. He listened to my symptoms and told me to meet him at the hospital emergency department immediately. There, he performed an internal examination, screwed up his nose and recoiled.

'Can you smell that?' he asked.

'I can't smell anything,' I replied dopily, trying not to faint again. I was feeling pretty rotten anyway, but to be told I also smelled rotten sure didn't make me feel any better.

There was an infection inside me and it turns out I was in 'cervical shock' (parasympathetic stimulation caused by products in the cervix leading to hypotension and bradycardia) due to pregnancy matter being left inside me during the quick curette he performed. My body was producing clots the size of tennis balls and was trying to pass them through my cervix. So, at the same time as I had an infection making me horribly ill, I was in enormous pain from clots trying to birth themselves.

But just like last time, it wasn't as simple as going up to a room and having that emergency D&C to fix the issue. It was Christmas and apparently there was no room at the inn. (I'm not ruling out the possibility of me being the Virgin Mary.) Not a single hospital bed was available so I was told to go home, pack a bag and meet the doctor at a hospital on the other side of town. Jessie drove me and stayed with me until I was settled, because Matt had to stay home with the kids.

By that time, it was late, so my second curette to get rid of the clots and any excess pregnancy matter was scheduled for the morning. It had been three weeks since I found out my baby was dead and it looked like I would be living through this pregnancy loss even longer.

After quite a few delays and a lot of, 'Well it's a *very* busy time of the year', the remainder of my pregnancy was removed. It was over.

Christmas came and went, the new year started, and my body

returned to normal. That's the weirdest thing about a pregnancy loss, I reckon. Your body returns to its usual state and the cycle starts again. The first period after a loss is a bit of a blood bath, but apart from that, everything is business as usual. Except your heart. That remains broken.

I had another early pregnancy loss in the first part of the year and a few months later, we stopped trying for a bit. So of course, I fell pregnant. I went back to that same obstetrician (the one who said I smelled bad) and he apologised for the cock-up with the curette and said he felt confident about this one, so I felt confident too.

Now, in between pregnancies, I had been doing some googling and investigating, and I had also been speaking to lots of women who had endured pregnancy loss. I had some ideas for how I could tackle the next one. I asked him if I could try all the things Doctor Google and my endo friendos with fertility issues had suggested, like steroids, low-dose aspirin, and progesterone pessaries. But he said it was looking good, 'so let's just see how it goes'. (I feel like you can predict where we're going here.) My hormones were rising steadily, I was feeling sick, everything seemed okay, but I still felt like I should have been doing something extra as a safety net, because I'd had so many losses. The doctor disagreed.

Just in case you were wondering why this doctor doesn't have a fun name like Dr Ned Kelly, Dr Eye-Roll and Dr iPad, it's because I can't find anything to laugh about in this whole situation, which is very unlike me. This guy does not deserve a whimsical name. Dr Voldemort is the only name that might suit, because he became 'He Who Must Not Be Named'.

At the ten-week scan, it was time for Dr Voldemort to deliver The News. The nurse said she had a good feeling about it, we felt good, but the big old scanning machine had other ideas again and the doctor sang that old, familiar tune.

'I'm sorry. This is not a viable pregnancy.'

We cried. Again.

Then he looked me straight in the eye and asked, 'When are you going to stop doing this to yourself?'

I had already been blaming myself every single day, and this question really sealed the deal. Words are powerful things. I wanted to shout at him, 'I told you to let me take the progesterone! And the aspirin and steroids! Why didn't you just let me try? Why didn't you listen? It might have worked!' But I just shut my mouth and walked away: another loss, another broken heart.

Fuck you, Dr Voldemort. Fuck you.

What not to say

When someone endures a pregnancy loss, it's really hard to know what to say to them. It can be confronting, uncomfortable, and downright awkward. After many, many losses, I have a pretty solid collection of unsolicited advice and unhelpful comments to share with you. The majority of people are lovely and supportive, but it's way funnier to share the shitty things people say.

So here are some of my greatest hits:

- At least you're doing your bit for population growth.
- Perhaps you and your husband just aren't biologically compatible.
- Have you thought that maybe it's your weight?
- My god, if you want children so badly, have one of mine. I have four. (– A nurse straight after I'd had a curette).
- It must feel awful that his ex-wife gave him children but you can't. (– An IVF counsellor).
- At least you have stepchildren.
- Stop stressing and stop trying and it will happen. (Easier said than done and not at all helpful.)
- Have you tried: yoga, acupuncture, Chinese medicine, meditation, oils, exorcism, etc.
- At least it was over quickly/at least it wasn't stillborn. (Whether

it's a loss at eight weeks, ten weeks, twenty weeks or beyond, no one should ever have their experience discounted like this. Don't do that.)

- I was so worried I was going to miscarry with my pregnancy. It was so scary. (Yeah, but you didn't, so this is hurtful and not helpful.)
- At least you can start drinking again. (I mean yeah, that's actually, probably quite helpful.)

What to do to help someone dealing with pregnancy loss:

1. If they want to see you, go over to their place with food, wine, tea, treats, and see what they're feeling up to. (Read the room, though. They might not be up to seeing people yet.)
2. Warm up a wheat bag for them, because the cramps can be pretty bad.
3. Give them something to watch, whether it's your favourite feel-good film or streaming suggestions. (Be careful of the content though – if it's about babies or loss, it can be triggering. I like to stick to action adventures because they're quite often entertaining and don't require much brain power.)
4. If you don't know what to say, just say, 'I'm sorry. That's shit. I wish this wasn't happening to you.' We know you mean well, but this is so much better than placating with unsolicited advice or accidentally insensitive suggestions. (See previous page.) Or you can even just say, 'I don't know what to say. I'm really sorry'.
5. If you are pregnant, give your friends who've suffered pregnancy loss a heads-up before you announce on social media, so they can be prepared.
6. Please don't stop inviting us to your baby showers and kids' birthdays – but don't be offended if we don't come. We'll be there if we can.

How to be sensitive to pregnancy loss

My mate Sarah and I are loss buddies. We have seen each other through a few miscarriages and we used to joke about having a Miscarriage Bingo Card. Each time she would go to a family event, she'd message me to tell me how many squares she checked off on her bingo card. A relative might tell her to try keto to stop her miscarriages, or an enthusiastic cousin might say, 'Hold my baby and the good luck will rub off onto you!' It's given us years of laughs.

If you haven't had a loss, but you want to be sensitive to those who have, try to be aware that the joy and excitement the person felt when they first saw that positive pregnancy test – all the planning, dreaming and imagining they were doing – has just gone up in smoke.

If you fall pregnant but you don't know how to tell us because you are worried about upsetting us, please don't block us out or shock us with the news. I know I really appreciate a heads-up if one of my close friends is going to bust out a pregnancy announcement. If they send me a message on the down-low before their big social media reveal, I am super grateful. I want to be happy for them, and I *am* happy for them, but I am realistic and it hurts like hell. So it's easier to process if we find out from you, rather than your Facebook wall or a staff meeting, or announced at a public/family event.

And on that note, this may just be me, but ultrasounds are incredibly triggering. I've had a lot of ultrasounds and they have all been dead babies (sorry), so when you post your ultrasound as your profile picture, I will mute or unfollow you to keep myself safe. I still love you, I just can't look at it.

Having a pregnancy loss when everyone else around you is popping out babies left, right and centre is quite isolating. But losing you as a friend is worse. We have just lost our baby. We don't want to lose you, too.

I know my situation makes people uncomfortable, especially

when they are making their pregnancy announcements and having their baby showers, but remember, as uncomfortable as you are, at least you get a baby at the end of it. Please don't stop inviting us to your baby showers and kids' birthdays, but don't be mad if we don't come. It might just be too much for us and we don't want to bring the mood down – but if we can be there, we'll be the best Cool Aunty you could hope for.

For me, Christmas is hard and Mother's Day is pretty much impossible, especially as people tend to use those times for pregnancy announcements. And if you haven't seen extended family in a while, often there are several new babies at these annual events. It takes a huge amount of courage and effort to hold my head high at these things and that can be pretty exhausting. I dare say there are many like me who will choose to clean up, do the dishes, hang in the kitchen, or get drunk with the uncles. Please forgive us. But also let us do whatever we need to be okay.

My fertility journey, continued

Okay, lecture over. Let's get back to the journey of fertility. I think we might be up to Pregnancy Loss Number Seven, another early miscarriage, then another. After that, I found myself up the duff again. By this stage, though, I had joined the board of Pelvic Pain Foundation Australia (PPFA), and the Australian Coalition for Endometriosis (ACE), where I found friends like QENDO President Jess Taylor, PPFA Chair Dr Susan Evans, and ACE member Professor Louise Hull. These women gave some stellar advice and direction, with Louise bringing me in immediately for blood tests. It was exciting having such impressive women as part of my cheer squad. I felt good. I felt confident. Unfortunately it was not meant to be.

Louise called me while I was watching Niamh play footy.

'Your hormone levels aren't rising quickly enough for my liking,' she said evenly and gently. 'I think this is ectopic. Are you able to get yourself to emergency immediately? I am so sorry. I will call ahead to the hospital and make sure they know you're coming.' She talked me through what would happen next and let me know she was on call if I had any questions or concerns.

I want to take a moment to talk about words and tone. Louise was plain with me. And while she was genuinely disappointed for me, she knew how distressed I would be, so she told me exactly what to do, how to do it and what was happening. After she talked me through what was going on, I was able to wait for Niamh's footy game to end, cheer as she kicked a couple of goals and then bundle the girls up into the car and calmly explain what was happening, just as Louise had explained it to me. There was no, 'it might be okay' or hushed whispers, just real talk. Maybe it was because it wasn't my first rodeo, maybe because her calm and matter-of-fact words were able to cut through the shock and sink in so I could safely get to the hospital, but I wasn't angry or panicked. It just felt urgent. But, being treated with a high level of respect and dignity made the whole tragedy far easier to navigate.

When I arrived at the hospital I felt sick, sad, surprised and utterly devastated. *Not again!* I thought. *I was in such good hands! How could this happen?* But Louise was right. My baby was growing in my right tube. I received a formal scan that showed me where it was and also showed I had adenomyosis. (To remind you: adenomyosis occurs when the endometrial tissue that normally lines the uterus grows into its muscular wall.) The hospital gave me two options: have both tubes surgically removed, or take Methotrexate. As mentioned earlier, Methotrexate is a chemotherapy drug, used to treat cancer, autoimmune diseases, ectopic pregnancies, and for medical abortions. I was not in any state to make decisions. I wanted my tubes removed because I wanted to stop miscarrying (you can probably see by now there is a theme of catastrophic thinking in my trauma responses). But Matt wanted me to take the methotrexate because he didn't want me to have another surgery.

I called Louise to ask her advice. I also called Susan. Both offered me their thoughts and took me through the pros and cons for both options. I often think about how fortunate I am to have had these two people in my life who were able to give me guidance. That's why it's so important to surround yourself with people who have the knowledge and skills to support you, and why I think choosing a doctor you feel comfortable enough with to ask embarrassing (or not) questions is key.

I chose the Methotrexate in the end. I spent a few days in hospital, then had to return every day to have my blood tested, to make sure my hormones were returning to base and the pregnancy was disappearing. This was one of my worst pregnancy loss experiences. The pain and the loss were awful, but mostly I was tired. So tired. Tired of grieving, tired of getting my hopes up and tired of hurting.

This tubal ectopic was also confronting because I'd had surgery and 'natural' passing through of pregnancies, but this was really different. I was frightened. Each night I said goodbye to my family before I fell asleep because I wasn't sure if I was going to wake up in the morning, I felt that sick. I only shared this with Matt after I'd recovered. When I heard myself say it, I sounded ridiculous and dramatic, but I think the cumulative trauma and grief – as well as fear of the unknown – had a huge impact.

While recovering from that ectopic pregnancy, I fell pregnant twice more and lost both pregnancies. And that was ten. Ten pregnancies. Ten losses. Ten chances. Ten heartbreaks.

After pregnancy loss number ten, I slowed down a bit. Ten was just too round a number for me to process in my head. It was like I'd filled my miscarriage loyalty card with stamps, only I didn't get a free baby reward at the end of it. We had a crack at IVF a few months after Number Ten, but I couldn't make it past the hormone blockers. (The first step in IVF treatment.) I'd just had enough. My body had been through hell and I just couldn't do it. I figured one of three things might happen: it would be the most expensive pregnancy loss I've ever had, it could kill me (by being ectopic, a fall downstairs or some other random complication), or I might have a baby. I didn't like those odds and luckily neither did Matt. When I told him and the kids I didn't want to continue with IVF, they were so relieved, and instead we poured our time and energy into becoming foster carers. I am now focused on the kids in our home and trying to let go of the kids that could have been.

(Not so) fun fact: I lost another pregnancy while writing this book. It was quick and it was painful and it has changed the way I initially ended this chapter. You see, I have always wanted to have a baby, so I didn't really want to end this chapter – both literally and figuratively – so my original ending had me leaving this on a cliff-hanger, with my hope still dangling. But it's time to let go. I always kept the faith and remained hopeful that one day it would happen for me. But now that hope is gone. Maybe I won't birth a child, but I have been so lucky to have been a teacher to hundreds of phenomenal, inspiring, cheeky, clever, funny, talented and wonderful young people. I am stepmum to two of the most fabulously intelligent, charismatic, unique and brave girls. And now, as foster carers, we get to love the most delightful little boy.

Normalise talking about pregnancy loss

I think the crucial lesson for me from all of this is that we need to normalise talking about pregnancy loss. It's such a taboo topic – and yet Australian statistics show one in four pregnancies end in loss. Why don't we talk about it? The most supported I ever felt with a pregnancy loss was when I was able to talk person-to-person with my doctor, ask questions and get answers, no matter how hard they were to hear. No hushed tones, no whispers, no unsolicited advice.

If we normalise talking about it, then perhaps we who grieve can feel less uncomfortable when people share their pregnancy news. We can better support people when they're going through a loss. And we can eradicate that shame and guilt that is so damaging.

We should all be holding each other up. You're not alone if you're going through fertility issues, or having recurrent pregnancy loss, or any other baby-related stresses.

I'm listening. I hear you. I see you.

13
Endo Education

early intervention and learning with
pain

Around half a million people who menstruate in Australia live with endometriosis. Two thirds of those experiencing symptoms are teenagers. That's probably not very shocking, because many of us started our periods in our teens.

But did you know, a Canberra study revealed that a quarter of teenage people who menstruate missed school because of their period? Or that of those, two per cent said they took time off school with every single period? So, let's say a person starts suffering painful periods in year nine and takes two days off school every month. Over the course of their schooling, that's around eighty days away from school.

School with endo pain: my story

School for people is hard with pain. From the stairs you have to climb up and down to get to your lessons, to the compulsory physical education lessons and sports days. And then there's some teachers' instinctive suspicion that you might be trying to get out of lessons because you're a teenager and therefore up to mischief. When I was in middle school, I was off sick a lot because I was exhausted and my immune system is weak. I catch everything very easily, from chronic sinusitis to gastro tonsillitis. (That's not a real thing, but it rhymes, which is fun.) I was constantly clutching a tissue or taking a course of antibiotics. I'm highly skilled at catching interesting illnesses: remember, I had malaria when I was five and lived in Papua New Guinea.

One of the problems with being absent a lot in upper primary and middle school is that if, like me, you were part of a group of friends with a culture of ganging up and excluding each other, if you're not at school to defend yourself, the person they pick on is you. Luckily my family moved from Canberra to Adelaide when I was fourteen years old, so I had an opportunity to start afresh. This allowed me to reinvent myself and be tougher.

It was the '90s, which was an excellent time to write angsty love poetry, crush on all the silly, floppy-haired boys, and listen to power ballads. I was an absolute drama nerd and had been performing from when I was five years old. I realised my teenage self was desperate to be a performer and a writer. I wanted to be a star. I could see myself on stage making people laugh, dancing, singing and then marrying Leonardo DiCaprio (because he would have noticed me at an awards ceremony that we were both attending and I would have cracked a joke that made him realise I was the most interesting, clever and charismatic girl in the room and we then would dance and kiss and get married on a beach under a full moon with a light rain). But I digress.

In senior school, I had a part-time job and was in all the school musicals. I joined the Rock 'n' Roll Eisteddfod, I had a lead role in the school production, I had a hectic social life and my grades were good. I joined a theatre company outside of school and I went along to any workshop, course or information session I could, to better my chances of becoming a performer.

But then I started to become tired. My immune system was failing again and my body just couldn't keep up with my ambition. My mood dipped. I started skipping school. Sometimes my parents knew about it, but most of the time they didn't. I was getting into trouble, not submitting my work, hanging out with the smokers on the hill (a superb bunch of beautiful scoundrels, some of whom I am still friendly with today).

And then, I just gave up. The more school I missed, the further behind I fell with my schoolwork and the more stressed I became, the more school I missed. This started to make me sad. (Cue more angsty teen poetry and power ballads.) I slipped under the radar and no one appeared to notice I was missing school every single week.

I discovered I loved earning money and being independent, so I took on a second part-time job. I worked at a pub, setting up the function room for weddings on weekend mornings, and by night I was a waitress at a fast-food pasta restaurant. Working was easier than school because there were fewer expectations and demands, and less pressure. The more I worked, the more school I missed.

Finally, my parents suggested I drop out of school and go to work full-time, so I did. My final school report revealed I'd missed an average of twenty-five days per school term. As a teacher now, I would never let any of my students slip away like that! When I notified the school I was leaving, I was required to go around to each of my teachers and have them sign a form releasing me from the grasp of the education system. Most of them happily obliged (and mostly wondering who the hell I was – they'd barely seen me!). But one teacher, Ms Zocchi, refused to sign the form unless I promised to go back and finish school when I was ready. I promised. And because I am a woman of my word, I did one better and sat the STAT (Special Tertiary Admissions Test), completed a teaching degree – and then actually went to work for her for a while when she became a principal.

But back then after leaving school, the relief was liberating. I was happier than I'd ever been. I felt like I could start accomplishing things and maybe even make my parents proud. I became a full-time waitress, but I was still getting sick all the time and I begged my doctor for help. He sent me to an ear, nose and throat specialist who ordered an immediate operation on my sinuses. That would fix me. To be fair, it fixed my sinuses, but not my low immune system, my fatigue, my low mood or my pain. But by then, I was eighteen, working in bars and living independently, so any doctor I visited said it must be back pain from carrying trays of cocktails, stacking chairs, working nights; and maybe I should quit my job. And, well, you know the rest. That was when I started blustering blindly through life, leaving a trail of misdiagnoses behind me.

Why schools should teach about what to expect with periods

Conversations about period pain start in school. I know this because I was a teacher – and I also used to be a teenager. And as someone who was diagnosed two decades after first presenting with symptoms, I am sure I would have benefitted from a program in schools to teach me about period pain. Not just a textbook explanation about periods and the menstrual system with pastel-coloured diagrams in a smelly, stained, well-worn science resource that people have scribbled penises on.

We don't talk enough about period pain and how many different levels there are. Or when it happens, and for how long, and what it's meant to feel like. Or why it happens. If I have lots of pain, am I normal? What about if I have none? The words *period pain* are unhelpful, too. It should be *period cramps*, because otherwise we are normalising pain. Period cramps should be uncomfortable, but they shouldn't interrupt your daily life.

By calling it period pain, we are allowing the world (ahem, men) to think that all pelvic pain is normal. But it isn't. According to Pelvic Pain Foundation of Australia, your period cramps are normal if 'the pain is only there on the first one or two days of your period, *and,* it goes away if you use the Pill or take period pain medications. If not, it is *not* normal.'[12] As you know, PPFA was the organisation I joined forces with to create a schools program, which has since gone national. They know their stuff!

I am forever grateful to have been part of creating something so useful and important for young people. And while I have now

---

12   Pelvic Pain Foundation of Australia, 2020 https://www.pelvicpain.org.au/period-pain/?v=ef10366317f4

moved on from the program and from the organisation, working on PPEP Talk® and presenting it in schools has been an absolute joy and one of my proudest life achievements to date.

I had the privilege of educating young people and teachers about period pain and endometriosis, as well as answering their many valid questions, talking to them about how they were feeling and improving their wellbeing by empowering them to know their bodies. But developing PPEP Talk® also educated me, because as I tackled questions from young people, I was finding out so much more about pain and menstrual health as we went along.

I have discovered so much about my own body, which has made a world of difference to the choices I've made with my treatment. It's given me the confidence and the language to ask for help when I need it. I'm far braver and more positive about my condition, which allows me to take more risks and do more of what I love. It has improved my wellbeing immensely. I still have pain and all the greatest hits of the endo symptom list, but I have a better appreciation for what everyone else is going through as well. I feel more supported, in better company and more prepared for what unpleasant surprises my uterus might throw at me. I am also able to help others and channel my energies into passing on the knowledge I have gained.

When I was younger, I didn't have the self-assurance to question a medical practitioner and I was far too embarrassed about periods and disengaged from school to ask a teacher. That's why readily available education and awareness about endometriosis is so crucial: it starts conversations and speaks on behalf of kids who are vulnerable, sometimes uninformed and probably quite confused, like I was. It also helps those, like me, who come from households where that pain was common, because the generations of women in the family may also have had the illness.

I've visited schools where I have delivered PPEP Talk® to groups of boys and male-identifying young people. They ask *so many questions!* They genuinely want to know stuff about periods. They pretend to be grossed out, but they're actually dying to know how it all works.

Without endo education, young people with pain could continue to be isolated, disengaged and disaffected. Being a kid with pain is hard, especially when the adults don't understand it either. I think back to my teen years. How often I was absent from school and how frustrated I became with being unable to do things.

I hated sports day and PE because I knew I'd be forced to do things that would hurt me. I got involved in theatre and music, but they would wipe me out with exhaustion. I would have further absences from lessons because I had to choose between my classes and the arts, or school and my casual job; I couldn't do both. I was so tired all the time.

I missed so many classes, hangouts and gossip in senior school; I would just move between groups and spark up conversations, or go home for lunch (and not come back). I was smoking, taking drugs and drinking because it seemed easier than trying to keep up with the high achievers – it was also self-medicating and I highly don't recommend it. The other kids had so much energy, while I was dragging my feet every day. I was also scatty, disorganised and distracted all of the time. Eventually I became completely disconnected and disengaged from school.

Now that I know I have endo, I can see from a distance what happens when someone is living with an invisible and often unexplained illness. It affects their involvement in school culture, social events and academic achievements. And their friendships can fail, which is heartbreaking for a young person.

Endo and friendships: Lucy, Chloe and Milly's stories

Lucy (sixteen) is still at school and has been struggling through friendship break-ups that she attributes to her endo condition. Diagnosed at fifteen, she has found the lack of understanding and awareness of her condition has driven friends away.

'My closest friend was horrible to me when my endo got much

worse,' she says. 'I was suffering constant pain, increased fatigue, anxiety and depression. I tried to lean on her for support by confiding in her about how I was going and about my appointments. She would respond weirdly and say stuff like, *Well you're seeing doctors though, so you're going to be fine*, or *you'll get better*. And I would disagree, because my doctors were telling me it wasn't going to be a quick recovery, and that made her just not talk to me, ignore me and exclude me from the rest of our friendship group.

'Eventually I distanced myself from her, but she continued to hurt me in class by saying stuff to me like *You're always sick!*, or *Wow! You're not dead!* if I came in late because of appointments, and just generally made "jokes" that were insulting, hurtful and rude.'

Lucy is learning how to deal with it by separating herself from people who don't support her and associating with people who do. I fully endorse her strong choice.

'I still have to be in many of their classes, but it's better for my mental health to mainly ignore them. It's sad, because I really loved my friend before all this.'

Chloe (nineteen) had a similar thing happen when she was at school. She lost a lot of friends when she was diagnosed at seventeen, but she had great support from her teachers.

'I lost ninety-five per cent of my high school friends when I was first diagnosed with endo. No one wanted to be around the sick girl and a lot of them questioned if my illness was genuine,' she says.

'I think being so young, yet being so debilitated by something you can't see, is a lot for your peers to fathom. How could they understand a concept when they have never heard of it or experienced it? It's naturally easier to avoid an uncomfortable or new topic. So I think with endometriosis being so taboo, they not only distanced themselves from it, but also me.

'I think they had a belief I was over-exaggerating my symptoms. How could someone who looks completely fine be in and out of hospital?' Chloe was told by some of her friends to *suck it up and take some Panadol*. She says she wished they'd asked her about it instead of making assumptions. She feels like her endo led to the end of a lot of her friendships. And that's awful, because she is such a sweet, bright young woman with an enormous amount of potential. I am confident she'll find friends and community outside of school who treat her with the respect and care she deserves.

Milly is twenty-one and was diagnosed at nineteen. She was bullied relentlessly as a result of her periods and she is still working through the aftermath of it.

'I started my period about when I was eleven. And it started out very heavy and hard from the get-go. I was very confused and shocked to find out that people didn't have debilitating pain and didn't have to constantly be at home,' she says. 'I was confused as to why none of my friends bled as much as me. And a lot of my friends didn't start their period in primary school, or if they did, it was just a one-day thing, or just spotting.'

'Birth control wasn't really doing anything. It was playing around with me, mixing up my periods, which would be three-and-a-half weeks out of the month, with maybe a two-day break and constantly heavy. I had so many stained clothes. There were some girls who had it out for me in high school, who once they knew about my bad periods would sneak up and say, "Oh Milly, you have blood on your dress. Quickly go to the front office" and I'd go and I would never have blood on my dress. It was really shit.'

What jerks! I remember being paranoid about having blood on me and constantly asking my friends to check the back of my dress and I would have been mortified if anyone had done that to me.

'When they first pointed out about my dress or tried to fool me into that, it was long before I was diagnosed. I remember they did it at the front of science class. They pulled me to the side to tell me I had blood on my dress and I ran, crying, to the front office thinking

Oh God, it's leaked everywhere' and the front office person would say, 'Honey, there's nothing there!' But I didn't understand why they would have lied to me,' Milly says.

'I was already self-conscious enough about it and it was my biggest nightmare to sit on one of those sweaty chairs during the day and possibly leave a shitshow behind me.'

Talking periods with young people in your life

Because periods are part of normal, everyday conversation in our house, Niamh and Keeley know it's not taboo and they can ask all the questions they want. Hopefully they will talk freely with their friends, which will have a flow-on effect (see what I did there?) and we can encourage healthy discussion about menstrual health, which can only have a positive impact on growth and wellbeing.

The girls are pretty good about me discussing the gross stuff like blood, discharge, poo and pain with them. I wish they hadn't had to witness my pain, but we've discussed in great detail what normal period cramps are and what isn't normal, and how to use paracetamol and ibuprofen, and use stretches to help ease muscles spasms.

I've stepped out of my comfort zone a lot since accepting my endo diagnosis, which seems odd, considering a chronic illness could have sent me straight into a very cosy couch comfort zone – where I could have stayed. But my desire to make sure no one had the same experiences as me made me brave.

Delivering the endo schools program, being in front of rooms full of twelve to sixteen year-olds as they ask honest, candid, graphic and important questions without fear, has allowed me to do the same. I am endlessly inspired by young people. I am passionate about arming my kids with as much knowledge as I can to help them to help themselves and help their friends. There is so much we can learn from each other every day.

7 tips for managing period and endo pain

1. Pelvic physio is a game-changer. Get around the stretches and treatment that can take away your pain when your muscles are spasming.

2. Your pain is not always related to endo lesions, but can also be your muscles spasming. So don't panic, thinking your endo has 'grown back' quickly after surgery. See above stretching recommendation. (But also see your doctor if you're worried.)

3. Diet can have an impact, so an anti-inflammatory diet is advisable.

4. Too many surgeries can be detrimental, so find a good specialist to work out a treatment and pain management plan that suits you. If they want to operate on you every year, they may not be doing you any favours.

5. Opioids are not a long-term solution. (I learned this after my surgery. The constipation alone makes my abdominal pain worse, let alone the fact opioids can lead to sensitisation of pain pathways, which make you more susceptible to painful stimuli, which makes your pain worse. Who wants that? No one!)

6. Treatments are not one-size-fits-all. Find something you are comfortable with and that suits your lifestyle and capacity. What works for others might not work for you, so don't be pushed into doing anything you don't want to do.

7. Everyone with endo has a different experience and no two cases are the same. That's probably why it's so difficult to diagnose.

14
Remotely Helpful

endo in regional and remote Australia

I have always lived in the city. (Apart from a brief three years of my childhood in Lae, Papua New Guinea, and a season working and living in the NSW snowfields.) From Canberra to Adelaide, then Manchester and back to Adelaide, I have had easy access to a health system that is definitely not accessible to everyone. Other than that time in Cooma when my appendix was removed due to my 'knickers being in a twist' (thanks, Ned), I've at least been able to choose from a range of specialists and doctors with varying degrees of experience.

But when I spoke with young people who live in the country about endo and period pain, they told me things like, 'There's one gynaecologist in town and he's my uncle, so I am not keen to talk to him about my periods'. Or that the local GP is their best mate's mum, so she didn't want to ask her for the Pill in case she told her mum. In one case, a girl was living alone with her father in a remote location, where she had to work on the land with him. She loves him so much and described him as a 'real country guy' who was salt of the earth, hardworking and 'very Aussie'. But she didn't feel like she could tell him about her painful periods – because it felt like a taboo subject, but also because she felt like she would be letting him down if he knew her 'lady problems' were interrupting the farm work she does with him. So where could she turn for help?

Online groups and digital platforms have been a huge help for many people, myself included. They're a wonderful support and if they're managed properly, they can be a wealth of information. But as they are often managed by patients and volunteers (myself included), they are not a substitute for qualified, trained medical help and advice. They're great to get stuff off your chest, complain about annoying endo symptoms and have a good laugh at this illness sometimes.

But sometimes when you're living in a rural location – whether it's your hometown or not – the challenges can seriously impact the effects of the condition. Or even worse, they can stop people from being diagnosed at all, due to the difficulty of accessing doctors, or financial strain.

Endo in Mount Isa: Michelle's story

Nutritionist and endo educator Michelle was twenty-four when she first presented with symptoms and twenty-nine when she was officially diagnosed. She was living in remote Queensland mining town Mount Isa (the traditional lands of the Kalkadoon and Indjilandji people, 1900 kilometers from Brisbane), for work. Mount Isa's population is less than 20,000.

'I'd just come off the oral contraceptive pill after taking it for a good decade (for acne and contraception). I wanted to lead a more natural lifestyle and opted to try the copper IUD for contraception. The copper IUD was an extremely painful experience for me, and I believe it was the triggering event that inflamed my endometriosis lesions that may have been lying dormant for all those years on the pill. After a few months, I had the IUD removed. Since then, my main symptoms have been deep, stabbing pain with sexual intercourse and pain with going to the toilet,' she said.

Michelle lived in Mount Isa for a year and a half during her toughest endo period. Just before moving to Mount Isa in 2017, she was seeing a gynaecologist in Brisbane who was about to do her first laparoscopy to diagnose her endometriosis, when she got pericarditis. Pericarditis is extremely painful; it's inflammation of the heart walls that feels like you are having a heart attack. It lasts for months and you cannot go under anaesthetic with this kind of heart condition. So her surgery was cancelled.

Despite her condition, Michelle relocated to Mount Isa for her dream job educating youths in nutritional health and wellbeing. But she knew she was in for a difficult time with her own health and wellbeing.

'I moved out to Mount Isa with chronic heart pain, worsened endo pain and not much hope after hearing about the services in the country,' she says. Mount Isa was very lucky at the time to have two permanent OB-GYNs in town, both specialising in obstetrics but with limited knowledge of endometriosis. After meeting with one of the gynaecologists multiple times without much success, Michelle decided against getting a laparoscopy with them. They used ablation as a method, not excision surgery. She says the hospital's equipment wasn't the most up-to-date and she'd heard a few horror stories.

'I just decided to go on the Pill and wait it out until we moved somewhere else,' she says.

It was too expensive to be flying back and forth to specialist appointments in Brisbane (approximately $1000 return flight). It was isolating suffering from endo symptoms and pericarditis when the local doctors knew next to nothing about how to treat either condition.

And Michelle didn't have access to any other specialists or allied health professionals, like pelvic health physiotherapists.

Two years later after relocating to Adelaide, Michelle was able to have her first laparoscopy and excision. While she still lives with difficult symptoms, she is now able to access a team of specialists, making her journey with endo much easier.

Treating endo in Bendigo: Dr Sarah Van Der Wal

Gynaecologist and obstetrician Dr Sarah Van Der Wal – who we've met a few times throughout the book – lives in Bendigo (located on the traditional lands of the Dja Dja Wurrung and the Taungurung Peoples of the Kulin Nation), and works both there and Echuca. Sarah has stage-four endometriosis, which allows a high level of empathy for their patients.

A town of around 100,000 people, Bendigo is around 150 kilometres from Melbourne. While the town is well equipped medically, there are some gaps.

'Bendigo is a regional centre. So, we have a fully functioning obs and gynae department. But at the same time, there's only ten of us in total. You can do a lot of continuity of care, which is really nice, because you can't get that outside of private in inner city. I've got chronic pain patients that I've been working with for years now, who see just me or trusted juniors. That relationship rapport is amazing. Some of the things that we've been able to achieve have been really, really wonderful,' Sarah says.

'But not having access to high-end ultrasound is a big deal; having to send people down to Melbourne for private ultrasounds is problematic. Our surgical waiting lists are actually lower in the regional centres, but you still get a lot of people for whom there's one doctor in town in their small country town that's male, so they don't talk to them about it, or they suffer for years. And then they come to you, and you have to wind all that back.

'And the financial burden on a lot of people in the country is very hefty when you can't access certain things, like tertiary-level ultrasound, or when people need that really expert surgery, because it's so far advanced they have to go to Melbourne for all these major surgeries, away from all their supports. I don't think the financial assistance from the government is particularly helpful,' Sarah says.

The financial strain for people with illness who are living in capital cities is stressful enough. In one week, I spent over $1000 on appointments and medications, which was a huge stretch. I got some of that back from Medicare, but only a small fraction. If I had to also pay for travel and accommodation on top of that, I wouldn't be able to treat my illness at all. Some endo patients can only work part-time. Others can't work at all, which puts an enormous strain on their illness, their family and their ability to take care of themselves.

And while the access to specialists in places like Bendigo may be more limited than city centres, it doesn't mean the quality of care is lesser.

'I think there's a bit of urbansplaining, where you get a lot of people assuming that if you work out in the country, then you must be an idiot,' Sarah says. 'Which is the most ridiculous thing, because we've got the same training they do, and we see everything, because it all walks through our door. It doesn't get diverted off to sub-specialists unless we divert it. But then we still do the work-up. We're working in Bendigo because of the access, and I have an extremely supportive department. I love Bendigo Health. I just think they're fabulous.'

'But the further out you go, places like Mildura and even Echuca where I work two days a week, the government hasn't funded outpatient services for gynaecology, which means that to keep the building, the hospital has to charge people. So, it's not possible for patients to go there. If they want to see someone for free, they have to go to Bendigo, which has a nine-month waiting list. And then they have to find the way to travel there, and cover the cost of the travel. It's around ninety kilometres, from Echuca to Bendigo, which means they don't get the IPTAAS [Isolated Patients Travel and Accommodation Assistance Scheme], because it's not one hundred kilometres.'

And, of course, that's assuming people drive. If they don't drive or don't have a vehicle, they are also cut off from many health services.

'We get a lot of people who struggle to get down, even to Bendigo, from the rural areas, and you certainly see things that have been left a lot longer than you'd like. I am very grateful to work in Bendigo but what we're missing is more of the advanced stuff that goes with a chronic disease. For proper physio, we have one pelvic floor physiotherapist specialist for 250,000 people, and she's overwhelmed. We have no chronic pain service. Unless you make it to the pelvic floor physio, there's no access to publicly funded psychologists, for what is a very life-altering, difficult diagnosis,' Sarah says.

'There's no real chronic pain department, no chronic pain clinics and all the non-surgical stuff like allied health or symptom management options are very poorly funded and missing.'

Rural and remote support for endo
What, then, can a person do if they're in a rural or remote location and needing support?

'You have a right to some investigation and that investigation may not show up anything, and you may not get the answer you want, but everyone has a right to it. I want everyone to know that they can advocate for themselves. If someone's saying, *No, I'm not going to send you to a gynaecologist*, but they're also not doing anything for your pain, then you have to sometimes walk out and find a different doctor,' Sarah says.

'And you just have to keep going until someone listens. It is not normal to have period pain that impacts your life. You should be able to get by with over-the-counter meds and a heat pack, and then move on with your life.

'And if you can't do that, then you deserve at least some attentive treatment and some attentive investigation. You have every right to advocate for yourself, at least demand a discussion with either a GP or a gynaecologist. I guess if I had any message for women, it's: if you think it's not normal, you can ask for a second or third opinion. If five doctors in a row tell you that something's completely normal, then it probably is.'

That's very good advice for us all, no matter where we live. This can be difficult in a rural or regional area if there aren't enough options available, but with telehealth, there should be some options for remote appointments and consultations so you can find treatment that suits you.

Advocates like Sarah in country areas are an enormous blessing and can mean a world of difference for people living with chronic pain. But because it's impossible to clone people – and Sarahs can be pretty rare – some patients are faced with an uphill climb on their way to a diagnosis or health care plan.

Endo in Yuroke: Kiera's story

Kiera has lived her whole life in Yuroke, Victoria, a bounded rural locality within Greater Melbourne, and first presented with endo symptoms at thirteen years old. It was the beginning of an eight-year journey for a formal diagnosis.

Now an adult, Kiera says she goes to the city to access care, but it was a frustrating time where she couldn't find a suitable health care team.

'My biggest challenge has been finding the right fit for me with GPs and specialists. Finding them over this side of town has been hard, as many are in the south-eastern areas. Being heard and believed was the hardest thing for me when I was younger. And now it's just trying to manage my debilitating pain as best we can. Living where I am is hard, as travelling is painful especially after a surgery and when it can take up to an hour in traffic it can make things harder,' she says.

'When I was thirteen and this all started, it was very difficult to find a GP who would take me seriously, or a gynaecologist who would believe me. It took until I was twenty-one to have a laparoscopic surgery and when I woke, my gynaecologist was crying. She said she'd never seen someone so young absolutely riddled with it.'

Since then, things have changed for Kiera and her health is better managed. She is living with stage-four, recurrent endometriosis, polycystic ovarian syndrome (PCOS), fibromyalgia, interstitial cystitis, chronic pelvic pain, and pelvic instability. She had adenomyosis, but has had a hysterectomy, leaving her ovaries. The internet has also helped with finding support and guidance for her illness.

'Nowadays, it's much easier to get good care, as the city is about a half-hour drive if there is no traffic. Until recently, I'd also travel 40 minutes just to see a good GP, but I've now found one much closer and he is honestly the best GP I've ever had,' she says. 'I get a lot of information through online research, appointments and online chat groups as well.'

Growing up endo in Cairns: Donna Ciccia's story

When director Endometriosis Australia's Donna Ciccia first noticed her endo symptoms, she was living in the regional centre of Cairns (the traditional lands of the Yirrganydji people of the Djabugay language group of Far North Queensland).

'I remember being sixteen, and having really bad symptoms. I used to ride my bike about six kilometres to school. It was downhill to school, it was uphill home,' she says. 'My grandmother didn't live very far from Cairns High and I remember riding to her place, which is only a couple of kilometres from school, so I could get that far, and I was in extraordinary pain. My grandmother was not known for being a very empathetic woman, so the family was quite impressed that she used to sit there and rub my stomach for me, and organise hot packs.'

It was around the time she was in year twelve that tragedy struck in Donna's life. She said the aftermath meant she became hyper-resilient, which could have played a part in her not being diagnosed until fifteen years later.

'We'd all gone up to on the Atherton Tablelands (the traditional lands of the Djirrbal and Ngadjonji people of the Djirrbalngan language area) for a school leadership camp for year twelve. It was early in the year. I remember I had my period and we were on a lake, supposed to be doing all these water activities, and I'm trying to be normal with everyone else, and not get down with the migraines and the pain and all the rest of it,' she says.

'On the way back from that camp, after we all bonded, I was on the first bus. The second bus went off a cliff, and the third bus came across the accident. Eight students died, so I lost eight very good friends. There was no counselling in those days. I think we spent a lot of time in the staff room smoking and drinking with teachers, and everyone was decompressing. Who in year twelve goes to eight funerals? It was quite a horrific time.

'I did have PTSD and I don't remember all of it. I just remember bits and pieces of that time. That was the resilience building. Whether you wanted to or not, you had to be resilient. The day after the accident, I had to get on exactly the same bus I'd been on the day before coming down from the mountain, with exactly the same bus driver.

'All of those things, you just had to get on with. Like endometriosis. It wasn't something that we talked about or discussed; it just wasn't a thing. You bury it, you push it down, you just suck it up and just keep going.'

Donna is of my generation, so I completely empathise with her experience of not discussing taboo subjects and just getting on with it (because things could be worse). But we have both chosen to leave that in the past, to start advocating for and educating people about the illness so there's no more of that burying it down and pushing through when you could be receiving treatment.

Accessing endo help, wherever you are

Thanks to groups like Endometriosis Australia, there is much better access to information and support groups that are accessible to you, no matter how near or far you are.

Most states and territories in Australia have an endo support group working to make life easier for people with chronic illness.

If you need advice, recommendations, a place to vent or to feel less like you're alone in this illness, you can just head to your local online support group and enjoy being wrapped in the arms of a community who understand you. And they do some truly incredible stuff. I've listed some of the support websites at the end of the book.

QENDO (based on Yuggera Land) reaches right across Queensland, including rural and regional areas online in person, and through their phone lines (1800 ASK QENDO) and QENDO app.

'People in rural Queensland have a completely different set of issues. They can be quite isolated. When you have endo, you're around workmates, you're around a friend, you can be at friend groups that are person-to-person. But in the rural areas, it's a minimum one kilometre until you actually see your neighbour, so sometimes, you don't have that personal connection,' she says.

'People in rural communities are relying on GPs who are sometimes old-school, or so young that they're on a GP rotation. People can be affected by communities who aren't willing or ready to talk about this kind of stuff. We have so many patients in the rural communities that are too scared to speak out in the media. There's a real social issue out there that just comes with being a part of that community, and there's also another level of, *She'll be right. I've got to muster the cattle.* I was a country girl, so I know how different they are.'

Luckily things are starting to shift, particularly with access to the internet, online support groups, telehealth and tools like the QENDO app, EndoZone and other digital platforms that are being developed as I write this and beyond. The tide is turning as we are becoming more connected.

Even though we are kilometres apart, most of the support groups are only a click away. People with your condition are asking the same questions you are. There are no silly or unimportant questions, so ask them: either directly to an online support group, or post your question anonymously. I will guarantee someone out there is wondering the same thing you are.

15
Endo the Book

(and another excision)

Due to my sensitivities to hormones, I can't take the Pill, have an IUCD Mirena, the depo or a rod implant to stop my periods, to slow down the growth of endo. I can only manage my pain with pelvic physio and painkillers, and have an excision every few years. Which brings me to my third endo surgery, and the hospital bed from which I am writing this chapter.

I've been putting off having this surgery. My hormones always go a bit wild after having an endo excision and can take a while to plateau. I have been really struggling for about the past year with endo pain and muscle spasms, so it's definitely time to get a good clean-out.

In fact, I've been in so much pain, I've been unable to reach down to put my own pants on. I'm far too proud to allow Matt to dress me, so I have managed a specky strategy where I put my pants on the floor (I even do this with underwear) and shimmy into them bit by bit, because bending down to pull them up uses up all the energy and pain tolerance I need to get through the rest of the day. Either that or I go pantless and the neighbours complain. Jerks.

I've also been having migraines during ovulation, which can be traced back to hormone fluctuations. They've been so bad I have been fainting and vomiting every two weeks, which has caused significant interruption to my daily routine. So I need to do something about it. I suffered a migraine while I was reversing the car out of the driveway and I crashed into the side of the garage door, dislodging it from its hinges. I bashed the roller door back in with a mallet to fix it. Don't tell Matt.

Endo surgery 1 (with Dr iPad)

It's been almost four years since my last laparoscopy, and it was in 2014 that I had my first one (see chapter one), which ended up as an ablation done by Dr iPad. An ablation cauterises the endo lesions, while excision cuts them out. More surgeons use excision as a method now, because they can cut and remove the entire lesion.

I requested a week off work after my first laparoscopy because Dr iPad told me it would be a simple procedure and I'd be fit as a fiddle in no time (because he was sure he would find a perfectly healthy pelvis). But that was not the case. He ablated as much endo as he could and in the aftermath, it took weeks for the pain to stop and months for my hormones to settle.

I remember feeling unsettled and uncomfortable. But because I had just started teaching at a fancy private school, I told my manager and colleagues it would be a super simple and quick procedure. When I went back to work a few days post-surgery, which was way too early, I had to keep up the ruse, pretending I was feeling okay, even though I was really wobbly. I sat through about five hours of parent-teacher interviews, but that was kind of fun. I have no idea what I said about the students. I let the endone do the talking.

Endo surgery 2 (with Dr Sherlock)

In 2017, I had another excision. The surgery was extensive and recovery was significant. My pain and hormones took a while to settle, but the difference in my body once I had recovered was incredible. I didn't want to go back to Dr iPad again because he kept trying to push me to IVF and a hysterectomy and I wasn't ready for that. I also knew he'd left a fair amount of endo inside me because he didn't feel he could remove it without the assistance of a urologist and a colorectal surgeon. He had originally wanted to cut my ureters and put in a stent, but I wanted to see if another surgeon could do it without all of that drama. Due to the medical traumas I'd had to date, I was a little tentative about my new surgeon, but he came highly recommended by my team of fertility specialists.

I'd moved on from the fancy High Fee-Paying School and was freelancing by then. And the week I finished up a contract as a publicist with a major arts festival, I was packing for day surgery for my second endo investigation with my new doctor (we'll call him Dr Sherlock because he loves to investigate and solve endo crimes). Dr Sherlock is a skilled surgeon with a dry sense of humour. He means business and he likes a challenge. When I told him that Dr iPad had left endo on my ureters, his eyes lit up. He was keen to get in there and excise my endo demons.

Before that surgery, I constantly felt like my body was full of tight rubber bands that would snap if I moved. I could barely walk, even on a good day. I was tired all the time and I was in pain every day, but was pushing through with work, step-parenting and life commitments, which was making me worse. I was in a very vicious cycle. And because I am a total martyr (but probably more likely because I had normalised my pain and symptoms) I was pushing myself to my very limits.

The recovery from that second surgery was long and painful. It felt like my insides were on fire. My hormones didn't settle for months and I felt like I was walking around with a cheese grater inside me.

But once I healed, I felt absolutely amazing. After that, I started pelvic physio and all the things that give relief from the muscle spasms that cause the pain even after the endo has been removed. I was able to do this because I had met a bunch of endo friendos who gave me advice, recommendations and support.

Endo education is power

After the first endo surgery, I was discharged from hospital with no information about what I had or what I should be doing about it. Thanks to the internet and some interactions with clever and educated people, I was able to learn about my condition.

But it always makes me think about all of the people who were diagnosed before Google, who had to use the *Pears Medical Encyclopaedia*[13] or ask their GP for help in a time where reproductive health, other than babymaking, wasn't given as much consideration.

We had the *Pears Medical Encyclopaedia* at our place, like many families did in the '80s. Recently, for research and comedy purposes, I asked my mum if she still had it. By good fortune, it was still on her bookshelf! We had a look at some definitions and explanations together. Our version was published in 1977, which is the year I was born, so this book was a huge part of my upbringing. Here's a fun sample from a book we considered a reliable source of information. (Disclaimer: it is not. Please don't follow the advice of this book).

This snippet is from the section about periods and period pain, talking about PMS/PMT. Enjoy the last two lines:

> *Premenstrual tension is common and many women feel uncomfortable just before the period with pain, irritability, and a feeling of fullness. It can be dealt with either with hormones or by diuretics, for example hydrochlorothiazide, since water retention seems to play a major part in pre-menstrual tension. Tranquilizers and Vitamin A have also been used. Ordinary dysmenorrhoea resulting in painful periods is due to psychological reasons, for example feelings of resentment or anxiety about the menstrual function inculcated by a stupid mother. It usually goes away after the birth of the first child.*

---

13   Brown, J.A.C (M.B., B.Chir.), revised by A.M. Hastin Mennett, (M.A., F.R.C.S.), 'Pears Medical Encyclopaedia', Sphere Books Limited, London, UK, 1977

Is it any wonder people of a previous generation were misdiagnosed and misinformed? Mum and I had a good laugh about the above excerpt, but it also made us really think about the lack of knowledge we all had, and the amount of bullshit we were being fed back in the day.

Whether it's limited funding for research, lack of interest in certain areas of medicine, a general disregard for reproductive medicine, or the patriarchy, there's enough of us who were brought up with that rubbish, that we are now on a mission to change it. From doctors to researchers, endo patients and educators like me, we want to bust some myths and destigmatise menstrual health.

It would take me years more of medical gaslighting, shrugs and eyerolls before I got the courage to say *enough is enough* and take my health into my own hands. It took an ectopic pregnancy to really drive home the fact I was behaving like a ball in a pinball machine: bouncing from doctor to doctor and slipping through the cracks every time. I had no direction, no guidance (except for the *Pears Medical Encyclopaedia*).

Even after my first endo surgery in 2014, I felt like I was blindly wandering around, unsure where to turn for answers. But that's when I decided to toughen up. I look at younger people now who are so much braver than I ever was, like Jess, Chloe, Teagan, Jamila, Lewis, Milly and Lore. They are standing up for themselves, telling it as it is and getting shit done. I am endlessly impressed. But it took me a while to find that confidence.

After my second surgery in 2017, I was armed with knowledge and that knowledge was power. I felt confident to handle my illness. I asked questions before and after my surgery and got the answers I wanted. If I didn't understand the answers, I asked other people without feeling ashamed or like a silly girl who was 'highly strung'. After Excision Episode II, Dr Sherlock told me he'd removed all of the lesions and adhesions, even the ones Dr iPad couldn't get. He told me all of my organs were stuck together, particularly my ovaries, which is why ovulation was such an excruciating time of the month. He also told me the procedure should solve all my fertility issues. (Spoiler: it didn't, but he tried and I appreciate that.)

Endo surgery number 3 – armed with knowledge

So here I am, at a hospital in North Adelaide, Kaurna Yerta, waiting with my gown and pressure socks on, ready to go into theatre with Dr Sherlock to embark on Endo Surgery Episode Three.

It's your typical scene. Nurses ask lots of questions; I answer honestly (except for the one about my weight, but she sees through my lies). The gown shows my butt to the entire ward. My blood pressure has been taken and I am waiting now to be wheeled down to Dr Sherlock and his team, so they can give the old girl a clean-out.

I've been nervous about it because of the accumulated trauma from my pregnancy losses and my past hospital experiences. But I know I am in good hands and the hospital staff have all been utterly lovely. The nurse looking after me is chatting about how she had to give up netball because of a knee injury. We bond over our bodies stopping us from doing things we love. She makes me feel far more relaxed and ready to go under. She lets me tap away on my laptop until they call for me.

In the lead-up to this surgery, I have had my eleventh miscarriage and my beautiful, twelve-year-old cat, Lula, has been diagnosed with aggressive bone and lung cancer. I am dreading recovery because I know it will include the loss of my Lula, who I hope makes it through before I am home from surgery. I want to say goodbye to her, at least. Being away from her is making me anxious, but I know I will be home in the next few days and Matt will send me lots of photos of her in the interim.

It's time to get wheeled into theatre now. I'm sitting in my bed like I'm a sugar plum fairy in the Christmas pageant, ready to wave to all my adoring fans as I parade down to theatre.

In the interests of full disclosure, I have gone back and edited a large section of text that was written under the influence of anaesthetic, Fentanyl and Oxycodone. It was funny, but it was also quite ridiculous. I am feeling pretty great post-surgery though, which is probably also on account of the anaesthetic, Fentanyl and Oxycodone.

My pageant float was wheeled down into theatre, and we had a great laugh as my 'drivers' accidentally rammed me into a couple of walls and into a minor collision with their boss. By the time I reached the operating room, I was smiling my head off because we'd had such a giggle on the short trip to my surgery. I climbed up onto the operating bed, flashing my butt again, but no one cared, because a butt is just like a knee or a chin to them, I guess.

I am introduced to everyone in the theatre and Dr Sherlock starts to talk with me about my work with PPEP Talk® and my association with several other endo specialists who are also friends of his. Meanwhile the anaesthetist, who is the same one I had in 2017, chats easily with me and joins in the banter with Dr Sherlock as he puts in the cannula and prepares me for a big sleep. I have a moment of sadness as I realise this is how my sick cat will go shortly, as I know she is not long for this world. The nurse notices the slight change in my demeanour and starts to joke with me about the oxygen she is putting on my face. It's a party drug, she says, and I ask for a glow stick and a lollipop. We laugh. I feel better. I am in good hands.

As I am set to drift off, Dr Sherlock is still chatting with me and must have remembered our pre-op conversation where I mentioned I was writing this book. This is the same pre-op conversation where he asked if I wanted him to put in an IUCD during my surgery and when I explained why I didn't want one (PMDD, hormone sensitivity, really don't want it), he said, 'Okay. I respect that. You're coming from an informed position,' and I nearly fell off my chair.

'And how's the book going? What's it about again?' he asked as people busied themselves around me, preparing the room and me for the big event.

'It's about endo,' I say, sleepily. 'And you're all going to be in it. So don't fuck it up . . .' I hear them laughing as I slip away into an anaesthesia dream.

Next thing I know, I'm in recovery, where I am trying to act sober, like I used to as a teenager when my friends and I would sneak the Tia Maria from my parents' liquor cabinet when we'd have sleep-overs. I ask everyone's name. I inquire about the prognosis of all the people in beds next to me waking up from their procedures, as if I am an expert surgeon on my rounds demanding to know how all my patients are doing. The staff are all in Christmas scrubs. I tell them they look great. They decide it's time to take me back to my room and I am not sure if it's because I am faring so well that I'm getting an early mark or whether they just want me to shut up.

Back in my room I call Matt. I tell him I think they just put me to sleep and didn't actually perform any surgery on me because I feel so good. Like really good. *Soooooo gooooooood.* He tells me that maybe I am on some hardcore opioids and perhaps it's time to rest. My dad calls me. He has been in hospital as well, having a small, routine procedure, but he tells me he is eating a cheese sandwich. I've been fasting since the night before and now all I want in the whole world is a cheese sandwich. Matt comes in with a cheese sandwich and Cheezels. Bless him.

I'm clamped to the bed with leg massagers to help with circulation. The nurses buzz in and out to take my blood pressure and temperature. Everyone is so friendly and lovely, and I actually get plenty of rest. This is by far the best experience I have had in hospital.

Matt jokes it is because I threatened them with a chapter in my book, but I maintain it's down to a few things:

1.   I am educated about my condition.
2.   I know what I want and don't want for my body, and I am now confident in how to say it.

3.   I searched for, and found, a medical cheer squad who could answer my questions and respect my position.
4.   I trust in the expertise of my surgeon, because I know I am being treated by someone who is driven by the desire to solve medical mysteries and get to the bottom of any issues, and also he told me he respects my position.
5.   I threatened them with a chapter in my book.

Knowing our bodies

The more we know about our bodies, the better everything will be for us. We will notice things that shouldn't be there, like lumps or abnormalities. We will get more pleasure from everyday things. Sex is better when you know your own body, because you know what you like, what you don't like and what your limits are. (This is particularly important for endo friendos, because intercourse can be painful sometimes.)

But the more you know about your own body, the more comfortable you will be with the decisions and changes you might need to make about it, especially with chronic illness. It took me a long time to understand my limits and actually start listening to my body. It took me decades to trust and forgive myself for my body's failings and my lack of knowledge and confidence. I realise I am being evangelistic and a born-again armchair expert in bodily functions. But I wasted so much time ignoring, normalising, concealing and being unwittingly ignorant – at times wilfully ignorant – that by the time I reached a point where I could properly look after myself, I had already lived a lifetime of pain, illness, discomfort and misunderstanding.

Dr Sherlock came to see me in the morning and said I had a lot of adhesions, which he has taken care of. He also says that he has removed a large amount of stage-four endometriosis. He explains he compared photos of the 2017 excision and my 2020 pelvis. None of the endo had grown in the places he removed previously; it had grown in new places. This gives me hope that perhaps my next excision might be easier again. Endo has been removed from inside my bladder this time, which he said should help some of the pain I have been living with. He explained some other things about my surgery and gave me tips for recovery and asked when I'd like to go home.

'After lunch,' I said. 'I pay enough in private health insurance, I'm going to make sure I eat my body weight in jelly and custard before I leave here.'

He laughs and leaves. I feel amazing. My body feels surprisingly good, my incisions are clean. I feel as if two kilograms of concrete have been removed from my pelvis. I'm excited for my life ahead of me. I know it's not a cure, but I am confident I'll get a few years out of this one, as long as I keep up the pelvic physio, cut out the inflammatory food and beverages, and keep stretching out those muscles when they spasm.

Recovery, reflection and cat cuddling

Back at home, I sleep a lot and cuddle my sick cat. Friends bring flowers and chocolates. Niamh and Keeley watch movies with me. Christmas is coming, so we put up the tree and I am even well enough to do some shopping. Though of course I push it too hard and have to go home, spoon with a wheat bag and snuggle up to a suppository.

Two days before Christmas, we say goodbye to Lula. She can't walk anymore and, while she is still purring, cuddling and loving us, it's clear she is in too much pain. She can no longer eat or use her bowels. I am devastated. Losing her is an enormous loss to me. She has been such a support to me whenever I am ill and she has been my feline heatbag for so long. Whenever I have fainted, she's been the first by my side, nudging me gently with her little nose and sitting with me until I can get up. She is the most gentle, loving and kind-natured cat and I have adored her.

Lula was one of a huge litter of kittens from a stable-cat that a saddlery were giving away. I had driven past the shop on my way home from a tough day teaching at a youth detention centre. A sign out front read: FREE KITTEN WITH EVERY LITTER TRAY PURCHASED. It made me laugh, so I went back and joined a crowd of people who were lifting kittens out of the cardboard box they were piled into. There were kittens of every colour meowing, climbing, exploring. One by one, they were being taken home. But one little lady sat patiently and still in the bottom of the box. She looked up at me as if to ask, 'Is it time for us to go home now?'

For years, until I met Matt, I lived alone with Lula. She was the best company: chatty, cuddly and chilled. When Matt moved in, Lula wasn't happy with the arrangement and used to bite his toes in the night. After a few years, she grew to love him and the kids, but the kids loved her from the moment they met her. Losing Lula has been so hard. The pain she was in was hard to watch. I wanted to take the pain away from her, the way Matt always says he wants to take my pain away from me. I had never really seen it as clearly from someone else's perspective before now.

It must be so difficult to watch people with chronic illness, especially those for whom we have so much love.

But Excision Episode III has been a success and I am so pleased I finally had the surgery. The aftermath has been far easier than any other recovery. I know this is because I am taking care of myself. It's been easier on my family as well, and has allowed us to grieve for Lula in a way we wouldn't have been able to had I been ill after surgery.

Too many surgeries can be detrimental to your condition and I certainly don't want to have many more, because my hormones are currently on a rollercoaster that is not even a little bit fun for anyone in my household. I'm definitely not a perfect picture of health and I could certainly take better care of myself, but sometimes I just like a bit of gluten, wine, not stretching, and being a blob on the couch. But I know what I should be doing. So even when I'm not doing the right things, at least I know I could be doing better and I've found treatment plans that work for the most part.

Weeks into my recovery and I am feeling good, despite pushing it way too hard in the first weeks after my surgery, like going to Christmas parties and overdoing it with tasks like redecorating the spare room – though in my defence, the redecoration was for a good cause. We were setting up the room for a potential foster child who, now that we've met him and love him, is definitely worth overdoing it for. Also I think the Good Drugs took a while to wear off. I got back on track after a few weeks of good rest and writing this book (turns out it wasn't going to write itself after all). I can't take hormone treatments so I know my endo will come back in a couple of years. But with pelvic physio, an anti-inflammatory diet and knowing my limits, I'm going to keep out of surgery as long as possible.

At my follow-up appointment with Dr Sherlock, he told me the endo he removed was 'very active' and I have to say I am annoyed my endo was getting around more than I was. Seems pretty unfair. I'm picturing it dancing with furry rave pants circa 2001, with that glowstick and lollipop I wanted in surgery.

When I mentioned that my recovery had been an absolute breeze, he told me it was due to my positive attitude. But I reckon it's because he's magic. Either way, I would say that much of my relaxed recovery is due to my understanding of what's going on and the comfort in knowing there are things that help.

Prepping for surgery:

- Make a list of any questions you want to ask the surgeon or anaesthetist. Include any medications on that list so you can ask if it's okay to take them before surgery, and how you should use them in your recovery.
- Read any documentation you are sent or have someone go through it with you. You'll need to know if you need to do any bowel prep or fasting. If you don't do these things when you're meant to, your surgery might be delayed, so it's best to be informed.

- Make sure you are clear on any added fees, gaps or charges so there's no unpleasant surprises when you're recovering.
- Call your specialist and book in your follow-up appointment. Some doctors are pretty booked up, so this will help lessen the wait time in getting any results or asking burning questions.
- Organise time off from work. Depending on how much needs to be done in surgery, you might need more time off than you think. Don't be like me after my first surgery and go back after a week off, only to end up taking another three weeks due to the damage I did by overdoing it too soon. You will need rest and recovery time and space.
- Do some meal-prep, laundry and tidy-up (so you don't have to think about it when you're recovering) and organise for someone to help with kids and/or pets when you come home from surgery.
- Have a trusted friend, partner or family member drop you off, pick you up and stay with you for at least the first 24 hours.
- Have your care pack ready and waiting for you when you get home (meds, heat packs, water, treats etcetera).

What to pack:

- Your phone charger!
- Any medications you normally take.
- All the paperwork you filled out, as well as your Medicare card, health insurance card, health care card and some ID.
- Your fully charged phone (with game apps, podcast recommendations, or e-books to keep you company).
- Headphones or earbuds (if you're sharing a room, you'll thank me for this).
- A book or magazine in case you need to avoid device light/glare.
- Loose, comfy clothes for when you leave (nighties are great

if you're staying over – elastic waistbands can be sore on your surgery wounds).

- Undies – period undies are great in case you have any bleeding, discharge or bladder leakage. You should also bring pads. Hospital ones aren't the most comfortable.
- Comfy shoes – slip-ons or slippers are good.
- Toiletries like deodorant, shampoo and conditioner etc. You might not use them, but trust me, that first shower after surgery will feel so good if you have your stuff from home.
- Snacks (but ask nurses and doctors if you're allowed to have them).

Recovery tips:

- Take notes (or voice memo anything you remember from what the doctor says) if you're given any post-op instructions. Or, have someone else do the listening for you. Sometimes the anaesthetic hasn't worn off when you're given information and it can fall out of your head pretty fast.
- Ask your doctor for a pain management plan (including post op pain medications) and make sure you know how and when to use them.
- Ask your doctor who to call if you have any questions post-surgery. Sometimes it can feel daunting, and you need to know if your body is healing or if something is wrong. This peace of mind is important.
- When you get home, rest. You heard me, rest! Recover, sleep, take short walks when you can. But give yourself time and space to rest and heal.
- You might have some pain in your shoulders or upper back due to gas used in surgery. This is normal but call your doctor if you're worried. Use your heat pack to help ease this pain (but don't put a heat pack on your surgery wounds).

- Don't lift anything for a few weeks after your surgery. The general rule is not to lift anything more than five kilograms. You will definitely feel the negative effects if you lift something heavier than you should, so do yourself a favour and avoid it if you can.
- Don't be afraid to ask questions, or ask for help from online support groups, real life friends, family, your doctor, or even the hospital (if you're scared or worried about your pain or post-op symptoms).

Stay connected with community

My first two endo surgeries took longer to recover from, partly because I didn't know what to do or what to expect. I now know endometriosis very well. It is hard, incurable, chronic, and it can be lonely and it is frustrating. You have to change so much about your life.

But I also know it's not the end'o days. It's not even the end'o the road. There are things that can help ease the pain. There are medical cheer squads who will carry you. And your endo friendos have got your back (and your uterus).

We see you. We hear you. We believe you. We are here to help you, advocate for you, hold your hand, heat up your wheat bag, fill your hot water bottle and walk this chronic path with you. Don't lose sight. We've got you.

Endnotes

Resources around Australia

1   Endometriosis Australia www.endometriosisaustralia.org
2   QENDO www.qendo.org.au 24/7 Support line: 1800 ASK QENDO
3   Jean Hailes www.jeanhailes.org.au
4   EndoActive www.endoactive.org.au
5   Pelvic Pain Foundation Australia www.pelvicpain.org.au
6   Endo A.C.T www.endoact.org.au
7   Endometriosis WA www.endometriosiswa.org.au
8   EndoZone www.endozone.com.au
9   Imagendo www.imagendo.org.au

Acknowledgements

An enormous number of people helped in a variety of ways to put this book together and I owe them all a debt of gratitude. If you are a person who had anything to do with this book being created, thank you. Whether through being my cheer squad, talking me through ideas and issues, giving me synonyms for words like 'support' and 'important'; telling me to shut up and write another chapter; making me cups of tea to keep me at my laptop; inspiring me, motivating me; sharing information or resources with me; telling me I can do this, or telling me I can't do this, which made me do it out of spite – I am grateful to you.

Specifically, though. I want to thank my husband, Matt. My partner in life, love, art, music, parenting, business, and flat pack building. Matt has given me the strength, confidence and encouragement to achieve every goal I have ever set, even the slightly more ridiculous ones. My favourite enabler, Matt has always believed in me and will always help me find a way to execute one of my harebrained schemes. Thank you, Matt, for sharing your life and your family with me and for knowing I can do things even when I don't think I can. Thank you for helping me to trust myself, listen to my body and argue with a doctor after two decades of medical gaslighting and misdiagnosis. Then, when the endo diagnosis came, thank you for silencing my imposter syndrome and pushing me to spring into action. It was you who made me brave enough to fight. It was you who ensured it was heard in South Australian Parliament. And it was you who walked me through the ins and outs of advocacy and bureaucracy in a world I'd never imagined I'd ever be part of. Thank you never seems enough for what you've brought to my life.

My best girls, Niamh and Keeley, and my beautiful little boy: you have been a source of so much joy for me. I may not have been the one to give you life, but you give me life every single day, and you make me want to leave a better world for you.

Throughout the process of writing this book, I learned a lot about people, illness, disability, and relationships. Everyone who shared their stories and spoke with me did so with faith and generosity. I hope I have done your words justice. Thank you for taking the time to show me what it's like for you to live with endometriosis and for allowing me into your worlds. I would particularly like to offer my gratitude and respect to the people for whom it was difficult to discuss their experiences due to cultural, social, dysphoric or traumatic reasons. Thank you for your courage. Thank you for educating me. Your stories are some of the most important, because they belong to voices too often unheard.

I would like to also thank all of the people I interviewed for this book who told me I should be tested for ADHD. There were a few of you! Thanks to you, I am now medicated, so I look forward to chatting with you again and showing you how good I am now at not going off topic or on a completely different tangent. I can even finish an entire thought without jumping to the next one. It's a whole new world! Thanks for being brave enough to tell me something I didn't want to believe. You have helped me understand neurodivergence and how to accept people for their quirks and challenges, including mine.

To all the endo advocacy and support groups across the country: it's not an easy gig to speak for a community of tired, sick, chronic and incurable people, and most of you are doing this voluntarily or for a nominal wage. Thank you for speaking for us, acting on our behalf, and getting shit done. Thank you for staying in the game, even when it feels impossible. Thank you for applying for grants, making programs, creating resources, doing research, running focus groups, raising awareness, launching marketing campaigns, lobbying in parliament, writing to politicians, meeting with people week after week, and working damned hard to get mention of this illness on the table. Thanks for starting the conversation so people like me can write about it.

When I was first approached to write this book, the first person I called was writer, journalist and absolute powerhouse Ginger Gorman who gave me sound advice and encouragement, which I am so grateful for. Thank you to my writing community for keeping me on track and afloat. Kylie Maslen, Vanessa Jones, Anna Spargo-Ryan, Petra Starke and all my other writer friends who said, *you can do it* or *shut up and do it* or just asked, *are you actually doing it*? Thank you. I appreciate you. I would like to offer my gratitude to the late Ruth Starke, who gave me some solid, but gentle advice after reading the first chapter. Her words were invaluable and appreciated, even if I was completely overwhelmed by hearing advice from a writer I have long been a fan of and just gurgled something incoherent in reply.

Jo Case, I don't know how to thank you enough. I am so glad you came to see my silly Adelaide Fringe show on your second date with your now-husband. I am so pleased you wanted to listen to covers of seventies music hosted by me, a wannabe comedian who was giving away crap prizes to people who answered quiz questions I was making up on the spot. I don't know if it was the terrible vinyl record you won, or my kazoo solo, but somehow this experience made you think I could write a book. I am eternally grateful to you for your faith in me. Your gentle encouragement, kindness, endless patience and countless messages of, *don't stress, we've got time* even when we definitely didn't have time were very much appreciated. *You* are very much appreciated. I am so glad we met and I am very fortunate to now call you my friend.

A huge thank you to Wakefield Press for publishing my story

and for supporting emerging writers, especially neurodivergent, chronically ill writers like me. Thanks to the Wakefield team, especially Michael, Maddy, Poppy, Milly and, of course, Jo.

I was able to write this book and conduct all of my interviews and research thanks to the Independent Makers and Presenters grant from Arts South Australia of which I was a recipient in 2020. Thank you for investing in me and for giving me a chance to tell the stories of people from diverse communities across Australia. When I called in a panic wondering if I could even write such a thing as a grant application, I received some advice (with kindness) that kicked me into gear for the entire project: *You're a writer, just write it.* Thank you, Arts South Australia.

Amy Hourigan: my friend, you are the most patient, supportive and encouraging person. I am grateful for you every single day. Together, we survive and thrive through all the things we have in common: endo, neurodivergence, our forties, foster toddlers, teenagers, tweenagers, hormones (ours and our children's), running our businesses, and overthinking. You are my very best.

Much love and gratitude to all of the people involved in the cabaret show, Endo Days. My band: Sam, Dylby, Tina and Matt; and all the people who have built the show, including producing, musical direction, selling merch, working the bar, taking door sales, and making it possible for me to create the show, which helped me to shape this book. I know I have missed some people and for that I am sorry, but thank you to: Niamh, Keeley, Peta, Vicky, Amy E, Leila, Amy H, Marissa, Finn, Vanessa, Josh, Alex, Myf, Ant, Sarah H, Malt, Sarah B, Gluttony, Renew Adelaide, Eloise from TABOO Period Products (organic and fabulous!) and anyone who came along and shared their stories as an audience member.

Special thanks to The Honourable Katrine Hildyard MP for her unwavering encouragement, for being even more excited about this book than me (and I am very excited!), and getting the ball rolling on my endo advocacy in the first place.

To all the patient and attentive doctors, physios, GPs, specialists, allied health practitioners, nurses and every other medical professional listening, helping, supporting and believing us. We see you and we thank you.

Thanks to the gaslighty doctors for the lols and for motivating me to advocate for me and for us.

Finally, thank you to the one in nine. The battlers. The warriors. The people living every day with endo. Thank you for fighting. Thank you for giving up. Thank you for pushing through, and for resting. Thank you for showing up, and for flaking out. Thank you for surviving.

Wakefield Press is an independent publishing and
distribution company based in Adelaide, South Australia.
We love good stories and publish beautiful books.
To see our full range of books, please visit our website at
www.wakefieldpress.com.au
where all titles are available for purchase.
To keep up with our latest releases, news and events,
subscribe to our monthly newsletter.

Find us!

Facebook: www.facebook.com/wakefield.press
Twitter: www.twitter.com/wakefieldpress
Instagram: www.instagram.com/wakefieldpress

www.ingramcontent.com/pod-product-compliance
Lightning Source LLC
Chambersburg PA
CBHW051433270326
41935CB00018B/1808